Dairying

Using Science to Meet Consumers' Needs

Cover photograph
©Dave Armstrong. Roslin Institute (Edinburgh)

Dairying

Using Science to Meet Consumers' Needs

E Kebreab
JAN Mills
DE Beever

NOTTINGHAM
University Press

Nottingham University Press
Manor Farm, Main Street, Thrumpton
Nottingham NG11 0AX, United Kingdom
www.nup.com

NOTTINGHAM

First published 2004

British Library Cataloguing in Publication Data
Dairying: Using Science to Meet Consumers' Needs:
I Kebreab, E., II Mills, J.A.N., III Beever, D.E.

ISBN 1-897676-14-X

Disclaimer

Every reasonable effort has been made to ensure that the material in this book is true, correct, complete and appropriate at the time of writing. Nevertheless, the publishers and authors do not accept responsibility for any omission or error, or for any injury, damage, loss or financial consequences arising from the use of the book.

Typeset by Nottingham University Press, Nottingham
Printed and bound by Hobbs the Printers, Hampshire, England

CONTENTS

Preface vii

1. Review of dairy heifer rearing and its effect on performance, longevity, costs and farm income 1

   J. Margerison
   University of Plymouth, Seale Hayne

2. Physiological adaptations to milk production that affect fertility in high yielding dairy cows 37

   V. Taylor
   Royal Veterinary College, University of London

3. Metabolic consequences of increasing milk yield – revisiting Lorna 73

   C. Reynolds
   The Ohio State University, USA

4. Longevity 85

   D. Logue
   Scottish Agricultural College, Auchincruive, Ayr

5. Optimising milk composition 107

   A. Lock and K. Shingfield
   University of Nottingham, University of Reading

6. Using biotechnology for the production and enhancement of livestock feed 189

   G. Hartnell
   Monsanto Company, USA

7. Customers and consumers health 199

   A. Minihane
   University of Reading

Preface

Dairying in the UK faces considerable pressure from many sources. Low world prices for milk and overproduction continue to depress farm gate prices in and many dairy farmers are operating non-profitable businesses. There is growing concern over damage to the environment as agriculture is considered by many to be a serious source of pollution, with livestock production being a major focus for amelioration strategies. To this must be added the concerns over animal welfare, and the conditions under which human food is produced, as well as food safety, particularly relevant in the light of the various food scares experienced by this country in the last 10-15 years.

This publication, arising from a conference held at The University of Reading in September 2002, contains a series of invited papers plus some offered contributions that considered a series of issues relating to the production of milk suitable for the needs of the consumer. Managing dairy cows can have a major impact on overall profitability and several papers covered wide ranging topics including heifer rearing, fertility and the nutritional implications of low and high input systems, along with a detailed consideration of the importance of cow longevity. Opportunities for manipulating the composition of milk for improved human health were examined followed by other innovative contributions with respect to the role of rationing models to improve the nutritional management of dairy cows and the use of biotechnology for the production and enhancement of livestock feed. Finally the conference examined the role of the customer and linked this with a detailed consideration of opportunities for the development of niche products, including the production of milk from organic farms.

The conference provided an excellent forum for lively debate and it is hoped that some of the information provided in this publication as well as the discussions held at the conference will be of value to those engaged in dairy industry and allow them to shape a better future for dairy farmers and all involved in the milk industry.

David Beever
Director, Centre for Dairy Research
The University of Reading

1

A review of dairy heifer rearing and its effect on heifer performance, longevity, rearing costs and farm income

Jean K Margerison
University of Plymouth, Biological Sciences, Seale-Hayne, Ashburton Road, Devon TQ12 6NQ, UK

Longevity and culling

The length of time dairy heifers survive in a herd and longevity of dairy cattle, was found to decrease significantly between 1981 and 1992, with the average herd life of a dairy cow in the 1990's declined to 33 (± 0.38) months or 2.75 years (Durr, Monardes, Cue and Philpot, 1997). In the UK, 21 % of dairy heifers are culled during the first lactation (MDC, 1998) while in the EU 33.4 % of heifers complete only one lactation (Durr *et al.*, 1997). In the UK dairy herd 48 % of heifers complete three lactations (MDC, 2000), while in the EU as a whole only 17 % of heifers remain in the herd for their third lactation (Durr *et al.*, 1997). In terms of culling of animals from the dairy herd, cows are more frequently culled due to poor reproductive performance followed by high somatic cell count levels and lameness (Esslemont, 1998). Most notably, reproductive performance has in fact become an increasing problem in dairy cattle over the last 10 years (Royal, Wooliams, and Flint, 2002; Royal, Darwash, Flint, Webb, Wooliams, Lamming, 2000). In sharp contrast, during the first lactation heifers are culled in decreasing order of importance due to; low milk yield, poor reproductive performance followed by mastitis and lameness (Durr *et al.*, 1997). It was clear that milk yield was the most frequent reason for which milk producers culled heifers and that the majority of milk producers did not use information regarding parental genetics when they made the decision to cull heifers from the dairy herd (Radke *et al.*, 2000). As a consequence, factors that affect the dairy heifer's ability to express their genetic potential to yield milk are of the greatest importance in reducing heifer culling rates and are likely to have the most impact on increasing the longevity of dairy cattle. Clearly, reducing the culling rate of dairy heifers would be both more efficient and ethical, but some consideration must also be given to what would be the optimal longevity for dairy cattle.

Economic evaluation of longevity

Net farm income and medium term net income

The net farm income (NI) and the medium term net income planning horizon (MTNI) were calculated using the lifetime records of 122,679 dairy cattle from 7557 herds that were obtained from Mid States Dairy Records Processing Centre (Ames, IA), (Jagannatha *et al.*, 1999). The fundamental heifer rearing costs including labour and breeding costs were included and longer herd life resulted in greater NI and MTNI and a herd life greater than 5 years increased farm profit and NI (Jagannatha *et al.*, 1999). In terms of rearing costs in Pennsylvanian dairy herds, the optimum rearing practice was not sensitive to seasonal variation in prices. The economic results per season of birth varied considerably, with the highest income per heifer being obtained from heifers born in December ($142/yr), whereas those born in May yielded the lowest ($100/yr) (Mourits, 2000). In addition, through the application of sensitivity analyses it was found that growth rate restrictions had a considerable influence and resulting in variation in reproductive performance and the expected net returns (Mourits, 2000). This raises the issue that restricting growth rates may not be appropriate for dairy heifers.

Production to herd life ratio

The relative economic value of production to herd life, which was assessed phenotypically on a standard deviation basis, was found to result in a ratio of 0.18:1 for NI and 0.46:1 for the MTNI planning horizon (Jagannatha *et al.*, 1999). Perhaps oddly, similar results have been found with beef cattle, where farm profit was found to be significantly greater when longevity increased up to 6 lactations in Austrian Simmental cows (Steinwidder *et al.*, 1999). While, increasing longevity beyond 6 lactations reduced farm profit, with NI decreasing when beef cattle completed between 6 to 9 finished lactations (Steinwidder *et al.*, 1999). These results may be considered irrelevant, but it is interesting that farm profits in both cases are based on milk and calf outputs set against rearing and production costs.

Sensitivity

In terms of sensitivity analysis, the value of milk yield sales in relation to herd life increased with high milk prices and low feed prices (Jagannatha *et al.*, 1999). While low cull cows prices in combination with high milk prices and feed costs had the effect of increasing the relative economic value of milk yield (Jagannatha *et al.*, 1999).

Longevity and net farm income

The average length of time dairy heifers survive in a herd or longevity of a dairy cow in the 1990's was 33 (± 0.38) months or 2.75 years (Durr *et al.*, 1997). Conversely, the greatest net dairy farm incomes have been associated with a herd life greater than 5 years (Jagannatha *et al.*, 1999). Therefore, it is clear that farm NI could be significantly increased by increasing the herd life and the number of completed lactations beyond those 2.75 presently being achieved in the dairy industry.

Enterprise resource utilisation

Individual dairy enterprises have a differing variety of resources and objectives, such that the most economical method of obtaining replacement heifers would only be determined by individual analysis of costs such as for feed, labour, health, reproduction, bedding, facilities, equipment, mortality and interest rates (Gabler *et al.*, 2000) or opportunity cost. However, in general during heifer rearing the feed costs incurred typically represent 60 (± 2) % of total costs, however no two dairy farms were found to be alike, with individual enterprises possessing differing abilities to control costs, rear replacement heifers and utilise critical information to improve profitability (Gabler *et al.*, 2000).

Reducing the culling rate of dairy heifers

Dairy heifers are culled at a rate of 33.4 % in the EU as a whole (Durr *et al.*, 1997) and 21 % in the UK (MDC, 1998). This clearly represents a great loss of replacement livestock when compared with the annual replacement rate for the whole herd, which has typically been approximately 25 to 30 % in the UK.

Figure 1. Culling rate according to lactation number in UK dairy cattle (MDC, 2000)

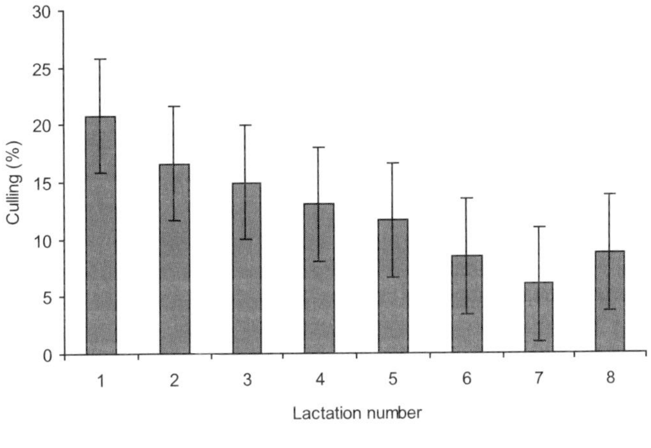

The culling of dairy heifers from the dairy herd during the first lactation was mainly due to low milk yield, followed by other factors such as poor reproductive performance, mastitis and lameness (Durr *et al.*, 1997). This was in sharp contrast to dairy cows. Thus any factors that reduce the ability of dairy heifers to express their genetic potential to yield adequate levels of milk during the first lactation are of great importance in both reducing the rate and increasing the efficiency of heifer culling. This should in turn increase the herd life or longevity of dairy cattle.

Colostrum

Colostrum provides immunoglobulins (Sangild, Fowden and Trahair, 2000; Davis and Drackley, 1998; NADIS, 1996; Quigley and Drewry, 1998), a source of energy and protein in particular energy (Baumrucker, Hadsell and Blum, 1994; Bühler, Hammon, Rossi and Blum, 1998; Hammon, Zanker and Blum, 2000; Hammon and Blum, 1999; Hammon and Blum, 1998; Rauprich *et al.* 2000a; Rauprich, Hammon and Blum, 2000b; Kühne, Hammon, Bruckmaier, Morel, Zbinden and Blum, 2000) and contributes to the development of the digestive tract, thus increasing the growth and development of the calf (Kühne, Hammon, Bruckmaier, Morel, Zbinden and Blum, 2000; Rauprich, Hammon and Blum, 2000 a,b).

Immune transfer

It has been well established that the ruminant placenta does not allow the transfer of maternal antibodies (Tizard, 2000). As a consequence, during the first 24h of life it has been established both legally and by farm assurance standards that calves must receive colostrum. This coincides with the permeability of the intestine to absorb intact the macromolecules and immune-bodies IgG, IgI and IgM, of particular importance was IgG, which enters the bloodstream (Sangild, Fowden and Trahair, 2000) to provide passive immunity and act locally in the intestine to prevent disease. The intake of colostrum has been found to impact on the parasitological and serological course of early Schistosoma mattheei infections. Calves, with significantly higher levels of IgG (H+L) and IgG, until day 73, to reach equal levels at necropsy, had significantly lower total worm counts, female worm counts and tissue egg counts and a 25 % reduction in cumulative faecal egg counts (Gabriel, De Bont, Phiri, Masuku, Riveau, Schacht, Billiouw and Vercruysse, 2002).

As a consequence, in the US, a plasma concentration of 10g of immunoglobulin G (IgG) per litre at 48h of age has been defined as a benchmark to indicate successful passive transfer (Davis and Drackley, 1998). While in the UK, the zinc sulphate turbidity (ZST) test has more frequently been used and a level of >20 ZST units was considered to indicate efficient passive transfer (NADIS, 1996). However, the efficiency of immune passive transfer been found to be affected by the timing of the initial feed, concentration of IgG and the total colostrum intake (Quigley and Drewry, 1998). The IgG content of colostrum has been found to reduce by 50% at each consecutive mechanical milking during the first 2 days postpartum and fell to < 2g/l after eight milkings (Levieux and Ollier, 1999). This indicates the necessity for colostrum to be consumed by the calf as soon as possible postpartum. The intake of adequate amounts of colostrum (4 l) with a high IgG (60 g/l) content allows the transfer of high levels of IgG into calf plasma (20.8 g/l) (Morin, McCoy and Hurley, 1997). To achieve the successful transfer of adequate levels of immunoglobulin, it has been recommended that calves should receive colostrum from multiparous cattle, as primiparous dairy cattle have been found to have low milk IgG concentrations in both Jersey and Holstein breeds (Quigley, Martin, Dowlen, Wallis and Lamar, 1994). This supports the theory that calves should receive colostrum of good quality, in adequate quantities as soon as possible following parturition (Drackley, 2000) and the importance of this has been stated in both the codes of practice (MAFF, 2002) and farm assurance scheme standards.

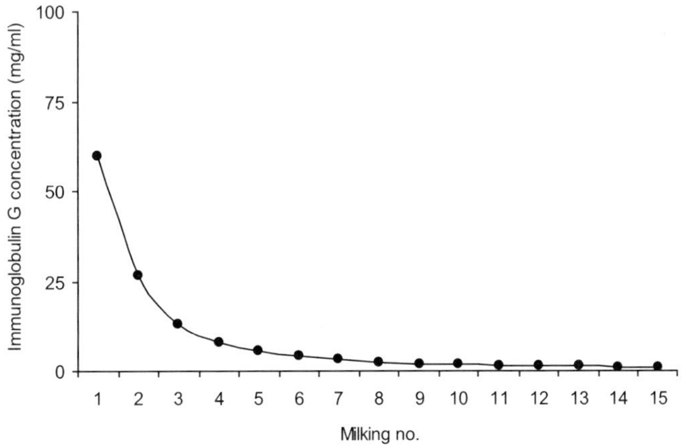

Figure 2. IgG concentrations of the first 16 milkings following parturition of 60 Holstein-Friesan cows (amended form Levieux and Ollier, 1999)

The use of computer-programmed automatic feeding stations has achieved similar calf growth rates during the first 3 weeks of life. However the plasma concentrations of total protein between days 1 to 28, immunoglobulin G, glucose and insulin at day 3 and insulin-like growth factor-1 at day 21 were lower compared with calves suckling colostrum from the dam (Schiessler, Nussbaum, Hammon and Blum, 2002).

Dried colostrum and whey protein concentrate have not been found to be successful in increasing passive plasma immune body levels (Grongnet, Dos Santos, Piot, and Toullec, 1996; Mee, O'Farrell, Reitsma and Mehra, 1996; Morin *et al.* 1997; Arthington, Cattell and Quigley, 2000a; Davenport, Quigley, Martin, Holt and Arthington, 2000; Morin *et al.*, 1997). Despite colostrum IgG levels being resistant to intestinal digestion and having the ability to maintain immune reactivity (Toullec, Lalles, Grongnet and Levieux, 2001). Grongnet, Dos Santos, Piot and Toullec (1995) considered that this may be the destruction or removal of specific absorption factors. Bovine serum derived products, seem to be more successful in the transfer of high levels of immunebodies (Quigley and Wolfe, 2003; Quigley, Fike, Egerton, Drewry and Arthington, 1998; Arthington, Cattell, Quigley, McCoy and Hurley, 2000b), these are however not legally permitted for use in ruminants under EU legislation. Further research is required to determine whether colostrum supplements benefit local immunity in the digestive tract.

Energy and protein content

Colostrum provides a source of energy and protein in particular energy (Baumrucker *et al.*, 1994; Bühler *et al.*, 1998; Hammon *et al.*, 2000; Hammon and Blum, 1999; Hammon and Blum, 1998; Rauprich *et al.* 2000a; Rauprich, Hammon and Blum, 2000b; Kühne *et al.*, 2000) containing three times more gross energy than milk on an as fed basis (Kühne *et al.*, 2000). In neonatal animals, energy has been found to be utilized to support glucose levels and maintain critical body temperature (Girard, 1986). However, the feeding of 10 to 13 l of colostrum during the first three days followed by the intake of whole milk has been found to result in growth rates of 250 to 500 g/d during the first week of life (Kühne *et al.*, 2000).

Table 1. Composition (/kg DM) of colostrum during first milking and milk

Component /kgDM	*Colostrum*	*Milk*	*Colostrum*		*Milk*
Dry matter (DM) (g/kg)	246	122			
Gross energy (MJ)	25.2	23.4			
Crude protein (g)	550	274	270	450	340
Crude fat (g)	256	273	350	470	380
Nitrogen-free-extract (g)	146	397			
	Kühne *et al.*, 2000		Roy et al., 1980		

Development of the digestive tract

More recently research has found that colostrum contains hormones, bioactive peptides, enzymes that play a major role in the development of the digestive tract thus increasing the growth and development of the of the calf (Kühne, Hammon, Bruckmaier, Morel, Zbinden and

Blum, 2000; Rauprich, Hammon and Blum, 2000a; Quigley, Martin, and Dowlen, 1995; Guilloteau, Le Huërou-Luron, Chayvialle, Toullec, Zabielski and Blum 1997; Hammon and Blum 1998; Rauprich *et al.* 2000a).

One of the non-nutritional substances that may be involved in the development of the digestive tract was IGF-1, which was present in higher concentrations from 313 ng/ml (Kühne *et al.*, 2000) and 512 to 1537 ng/ml (Baumrucker *et al.*, 1994) while IGF1 concentrations in milk are < 2 ng/ml (Kühne *et al.*, 2000). Specific receptors for both IGF-1 and IGF-2 have been found to exist in the intestinal mucosa (Baumrucker *et al.*, 1994). Colostrum providing 750 ng/ml of IGF-1 was found to stimulate the development of the intestinal villi, especially in the duodenum increasing the villi surface area 1.5 fold compared with calves fed milk substitute (Bühler *et al.*, 1998). The feeding of IGF-1 at 750 ng/ml of reconstituted milk substitute for one week was found to accelerate intestinal DNA synthesis and significantly increase [^{3}H] thymidine incorporation into duodenal, jujenal and ileal tissue (Baumrucker *et al.*, 1994), while the oral administration of IGF-1 did not increase DNA:protein ratio in intestinal tissue or stimulate intestinal morphological differentiation (Bühler *et al.*, 1998). Bühler *et al.* (1998) concluded that not only IGFs but other non-nutritional factors present in colostrum may contribute to the development of the digestive tract.

Hammon and Blum (1999) found that the intake of colostrum reduced plasma glutamine, which was a preferred source of nutrient for enterocytes, concentrations from 275-325 μmol/l at birth to 75-150 μmol/l at 24h of age. These calves also had a positive effect of colostrum on gut development and the rapid reduction in glutamine levels was probably associated with enhanced gut growth (Hammon and Blum, 1999). Calves receiving colostrum have higher plasma triglyceride concentrations, insulin responses to feeding and IGF-1 in blood plasma levels, carbohydrate absorptive capacity while formula fed calves had higher plasma glucagon levels which may indicate higher rates of gluconeogenesis in response to lower absorption of glucose and triglyceride (Rauprich *et al.*, 2000a).

Colostrum has been associated with the release of pancreatic enzymes, such as lipase (Le Huërou-Luron, Guilloteau, Wicker-Planquart, Chayvialle, Burton, Mouats, Toullec and Puigserver, 1992; Guilloteau, Chayvialle, Toullec, Grongent and Bernard (1992). These peptides may be implicated in the stimulation of pancreatic secretion (Guilloteau *et al.* 1997) and could complement those present in colostrum thus ensuring efficient digestion of nutrients, especially triglyceride (Rauprich *et al.* 2000a).

High feeding rates

More recently, studies have shown that young Holstein dairy calves can grow efficiently on a high feeding rate of milk substitute >900 g substitute /d (Diaz, Smith and Van Amburgh, 1998). This has relaunched a debate on appropriate quantity and composition of milk substitute for young calves, especially heifer replacements. The higher feeding rates of 800 – 1000g DM/d of milk substitute are much greater when compared with early weaning systems which use 450g DM/d of milk substitute. As a consequence, higher milk substitute feeding levels during the early life may have a positive effect on the development, health and lifetime profitability of the dairy herd (Troccon, 1993, Drackley, 2001a).

Disease control and prevention

Colostrum and pathogen challenge

Environmental conditions, pathogen pressure and management may interfere with the ability of colostrum to protect the calf from disease. Outbreaks of scour in the UK has occurred even in calves with adequate immunoglobulin levels, indicated by ZST level (NADIS, 1996). There are a number of factors that have been associated with scouring including wet bedding, group rearing, whole milk feeding, low frequency of building disinfection and compound feeding. In France and the UK the micro-organism most frequently encountered was rotavirus, associated with between 22.4 and 29% of the cases of scouring, followed by Cyptosporidium (16.9 to 20%), Coronavirus (6 to 6.3%), E.coli (4 to 7.5 %) and Salmonella (3 to 8 %). (Portejoie, 1997; NADIS, 1996) The importance of Cryptosporidium has been highlighted in a number of studies (Portejoie, 1997; Quigley *et al.*, 1995; NADIS, 1996). However, specific colostral antibodies are not always effective in protecting calves against disease challenges. In particular *C. parvum* (Harp, Woodmansee and Moon, 1989) and given the human health hazard of *C. parvum* in this case farm biosecurity was especially important.

The 'weak' period

This period has been found to occur mainly in the second and third weeks of life, when the level of maternal antibodies and transferred passive immunity decreases and the development of the active immunity did not have a fully developed response (Tizard, 2000). Thus the immune system of the calf was inadequate to provide an effective specific response to the infection. The majority of the reported incidences of scouring have been found to occur during this period (NADIS, 1996: Portejoie, 1997). During this period, the feeding and management strategies should stimulate the natural defence of the young calf and may involve the use of physical barriers, the addition of intestinal microflora and the development of an innate immunity, accelerating the maturity of the immune system. These factors should be encouraged by adequate colostrum intake and good environmental conditions.

Calves with significantly higher levels of IgG (H+L) and IgG, until day 73, to reach equal levels at necropsy had significantly lower total worm counts, female worm counts and tissue egg counts and a 25 % reduction in cumulative faecal egg counts (Gabriel, De Bont, Phiri, Masuku, Riveau, Schacht, Billiouw and Vercruysse, 2002).

Calf nutrition

Dairy heifer rearing systems

There are a number of different feeding systems and milk types that can be utilised in dairy heifer rearing programmes.

Feeding systems

Dairy heifer calves can be fed; twice daily from a bucket or pail, ad-libitum feeding of cold acidified milk, ad-libitum feeding warm milk substitute from a machine and even computer controlled feeding systems. In all of these feeding systems, the highest growth rates and lowest mortality have been achieved by feeding the milk substitute according to the manufacturer's instructions. In particular including the milk substitute at the correct concentration, mixing substitute thoroughly as this has been found to reduce the levels of diarrhoea and subsequent mortality. Finally, feeding milk substitute at the recommended temperature has been found to reduce possible breakdown of fat and degradation of protein quality due to possible de-naturing of amino acids caused by high temperatures.

Types of milk

The milk used can be either milk substitute, skim milk powder or zero skim powder, or whole milk which has typically been used in countries where milk quota restrictions are in place. The higher quality milk substitutes contain 50 to 60 % skimmed milk powder and when reconstituted the protein fraction of the milk forms into clots in the abomasum of the calf. This clotting reduces the rate of digestion, which reduces the incidence of diarrhoea and scouring, which has been found to be reduced even further with acidification of skim milk powder. As a consequence these milk substitutes are well suited to being fed from a bucket or pail or through a machine. The zero skim milk powder contains whey, concentrated whey protein along with vegetable proteins such as soya. These products do not form into clots in the abomasum and as a consequence are more suitable for frequent feeding by machine and when used in a twice daily feeding system the feeding of high levels of these to calves < 4 weeks of age should be avoided. The milk substitute mixing rates and temperature and the feeding temperature, amount fed per feed and per day of whole milk and milk substitutes in differing milk feeding systems are presented in Table 2.

Table 2. The milk replacer mixing rates and temperature, feeding temperature, amount fed per feed and per day in differing milk feeding systems

	Mixing		*Feeding*		
Feeding system	*Rate* (g/l)	*Temp.* (°C)	*Temp.* (°C)	*l/feed*	*l/calf/d*
Twice /d using bucket / pail					
Whole milk	-	-	0 - 36	2 - 3	4 - 6
Skim milk powder	125	40	36	2	4
Ad-libitum systems					
Cold acidified replacer	125	-		-	8
Warm milk from machine	100-125	20-40	20-40	-	8

Level of milk feeding

In the UK and EU (Tanan and Newbold, 2002) and the USA (Heinrichs, Well and Losinger 1995), the most common method of rearing dairy heifers has been to feed calves from a bucket twice daily with limited amounts of either whole milk or milk. This limiting of milk feeding encourages dry feed intake and 'early weaning' from which they take their name. These systems have been found to be less expensive per kg of liveweight gain compared with adlibitum feeding systems (Thickett *et al.* 1988), which require considerably greater levels of milk substitute. However, more recently in the US dairy heifer rearing has been undertaken using higher levels of milk substitute feeding during the prepubertal growth period and the systems are presently referred to as 'accelerated growth'. These systems have been found to increase feed conversion efficiency (Van Amburgh *et al*, 1998; Diaz *et al.*, 1998), calf health (Nonnecke *et al.*, 2000; Smith *et al.*, 2000) and reduce overall dairy replacement rearing costs by reducing age at first parturition (Mauritis at al., 1999 and 2000). These feed intake levels and growth rates are more like those found with natural suckling.

Milk feeding systems and prepubertal growth rates

Limited milk or milk substitute feeding and early weaning systems

The feeding of dairy heifers from a bucket twice daily has typically limited the amount milk substitute fed to approximately 11 g milk substitute DM/kg body weight (BW)/day). This has the effect of stimulating the intake of supplementary dry feed and increasing the rate of rumen development. These systems are designed to limit the amount of liquid milk utilised, increase the levels of supplementary dry feed used to encourage early weaning and subsequently reduce the milk level used and labour required to rear calves. These systems allow the calf to be weaned as early as 6 weeks, but more recently dairy calves are more typically weaned at approximately 8 weeks of age in conventional and 12 weeks of age in organic milk production systems. These 'early weaning' systems have been common practice in dairy enterprises in the EU, UK (Tanan and Newbold, 2002) and the USA (Heinrichs *et al.*, 1995). Unfortunately, dairy heifer rearing practices have been determined by short-term economic considerations, frequently based on data from rearing of beef cattle breeds rather than considering the long-term productivity of dairy heifers.

However, more recently it has been found that the rearing of dairy heifers begins with neonatal nutrition of the calf (Brown *et al.*, 2002) and possibly even the pregnant dairy cow. The nutrition of the dairy replacements has been found to have significant effects on the productivity of the dairy heifer with increased or accelerated growth rates increasing milk yield in dairy heifers (Troccon, 1993; Van Amburgh *et al*, 1998; NRC, 2001; Sejrsen and Purup, 1997; Knight, 2001) and thus longevity of the dairy cow. Typically, feeding levels have been restricted, but high levels of milk feeding and subsequently accelerated growth rates during the prepubertal phase are controversial.

Growth rates

Prepubertal growth rates and mammary development

In dairy replacement heifers, high levels of feeding resulting in high growth rates during the prepubertal period (approximately 3 months of age) when an allometric period of mammary development occurs has been associated with an increased deposition of fat in mammary parenchymal tissue (Sejrsen and Purup, 1997) reducing the long term milk production potential of dairy cattle. However, this effect has not consistently resulted in a decline in subsequent milk production (Sejrsen and Purup, 1997). The conflicting results are likely to be due to differences in growth being confounded by differences in body size at calving. The lower milk yield from heifers with higher prepubertal growth rates occurred in heifers that were 30kg lighter at calving compared with herdmates grown at lower rates (Van Amburgh *et al.*, 1998). Moreover, negative effects of high prepubertal growth rates on mammary development were not found when high levels of protein were supplied, 30 % CP (VandeHaar, 1997). In addition, the growth rate at which milk yield potential could be reduced may vary between breeds. In higher genetic merit dairy breeds, it was found to be approximately 700g/d (Sejrsen and Purup, 1997). While more recently no negative effects have been found when Holstein dairy heifers were grown at approximately 900g/d during the prepubertal period (Knight, 2001). In 2002 the NRC proposed a target pre-pubertal growth rate of 870g/d, which taking into consideration the contradictory nature of much of the research at that point seemed to be a sensible approach until further research has been completed.

Ad libitum milk and acidified milk substitute consumption

In 1968 Khouri and Pickering fed whole milk to calves during the first 6 weeks of life, at rates of 11.3%, 13.9%, 15.9%, or 19.4% of body weight and growth rates increased with increasing feeding rate at 404, 500, 623, and 941g/d, respectively. However, the feed conversion efficiency in kg milk DM per kg liveweight gain decreased with increasing feeding levels to 1.58, 1.48, 1.34, and 1.23, respectively (Khouri and Pickering, 1968). However, calves that suckled daily for 6 weeks, had higher growth rates 850g/d, compared with 560g/d in calves fed milk substitute calved at a younger age, had higher live weight at calving and greater first lactation yields compared (Bar-Peled, Robinson, Maltz, Tagari, Folman, Bruckental, Voet, Gacitua and Lehrer, 1997). Although it was not possible to isolate the direct cause of this extra milk production, the potential impact of calf nutrition on dairy cow performance was clearly an issue.

The research into the adlibitum consumption of acidified milk substitutes by calves was completed in the 1980's (Nocek and Braund, 1986; Richard *et al.*, 1998) and was reviewed by Davis and Drackley in 1998. Thickett *et al.* (1988) found that *ad libitum* feeding systems, in which intake levels were approximately 18-20g/kg BW as milk substitute DM, were approximately 0.24 more expensive per kg BWG than twice-daily bucket systems using approximately 10g/kg BW as milk substitute DM. It was not cost alone but the long-term efficiency of heifer rearing systems that should be considered. However, the rearing of dairy heifers for early calving at 24 months was identified some time ago as one situation where restricting milk substitute may not be appropriate (Thickett, Mitchell and Hallows, 1988). It seems at this point that neither this restriction nor adlibitum feeding of milk substitute fulfils the requirements of dairy heifer rearing.

Higher levels of milk substitute feeding has typically been found to reduce dry feed intake, delay rumen development and reduce the net increase in nutrient intake. The use of conventional milk substitute at a 1:1 ratio of CP:fat was found to reduce dry feed intake as feeding level increased which resulted in milk substitue feeding level having no effect on growth rate (Hill, Aldrich, Proeschel and Schlotterbeck, 2001). However, when the protein:fat ratio of the milk substitute was increased, increasing feeding level from 450g/d to 680g/d equivalent to approximately 10 to 15g/kg BW as milk substitute DM, had no effect on dry feed intake, while liveweight gain was increased (Hill *et al.*, 2001). In systems that involve high levels of liquid milk consumption, and where the protein:fat ratio has not been increased, it is important to ensure that dry feed intake levels are encouraged and are adequate to support growth rate prior to fully weaning calves from liquid milk consumption. In addition, experimental work is required to assess the interaction between milk substitute feeding level and protein concentration at a range of feeding levels.

Metabolic imprinting

In many species early malnutrition has been found to impede cell division to the extent that mature body size, defined as the point of maximum muscle mass, has been reduced (Owens, Dubeski and Hanson, 1993). This metabolic imprinting started with hyperplasia (cell multiplication) in young animals and progressively develops into cell enlargement (hypertrophy) as the animal develops. Despite the limited evidence of metabolic imprinting being available in dairy cattle. The hypothesis that sub-optimal nutrition of calves may have a long-term influence on the size of the body protein pool and possible effect on milk protein yield through the mobilisation of labile body protein reserves in dairy cattle remains a possibility. The possibility that nutritional status during the neonatal period may affect the animals ability to respond to hormones in adult dairy cattle was raised by Drackley (2000). However, as yet there is no evidence to support this.

Increased or 'accelerated' prepubertal growth

While a number of factors have driven this development, the main issue was the concern that traditional calf rearing practices which restrict milk feeding levels do not have sufficiently high live weight gain to allow heifers to calve at less than 24months of age. The increasing merit of dairy heifers and the increasing popularity of contract heifer rearing due to increasing herd size in response to economic constrains on milk producers has brought forward the need for changes in heifer growth rates. These so-called 'accelerated growth' programmes for dairy heifer calves have been developed in the USA from research completed by Van Amburgh and colleagues at Cornell University (Diaz *et al.*, 1998; Tikofsky *et al.*, 2001) and were reviewed recently by Drackley (2001 a, b) and Tannan and Newbold (2001).

In this system dairy heifers are fed much larger volumes of milk substitute to achieve growth rates of 1000 g during the first 5 wk of life (Diaz *et al.*, 1998). The deposition of fat was alleviated by the high protein content of the milk substitute i.e. 30% CP used in current research, which promoted lean growth and dairy heifers do not deposit fat within the mammary tissue. Accelerated growth has been found to have high feed conversion efficiency, probably due to the first 2 months of life being the most efficient period to increase stature (Kertz *et al.*, 1998) and increased immune function and calf health (Nonnecke *et al.*, 2000; Smith *et al.*, 1998). However, the greatest advantage of accelerated growth was the reduction in heifer rearing costs due to the decrease in time to breeding size and subsequent age at first calving.

Diaz *et al.* (2001) used high feeding rates and found that liveweight gain in calves fed 23.5g/kg BW as milk substitute DM with additional dry feeding had a lower protein:fat ratio than the liveweight gain in calves fed 14.3g/kg BW as milk substitute DM. While, Drackley (2001b) feeding dairy calves approximately 18g/kg BW as milk substitute DM found only slight increases in the fat content of body tissue. More data is required on effects of feeding level on skeletal growth such as liveweight, body composition, height at withers, hip width etc.

Effect of target breeding age and weight on growth rates

The target breeding weight was 390kg at 13.4mo of age Mourits (2000). Dairy calves, between breeding and 3 months of age heifers gain a maximum of 275kg (10.4mo at 850g/d) and thus they must be 115kg at 3mo of age, which with a birth weight of 40 to 45 kg, they should grow at 822g/d between 0 to 3 months. While in France, Troccon (1993) proposed that autumn-born calves should reach 0.30 (30%) of mature body weight by the end of the first winter approximately 6mo of age, which would require a growth rate of 850g/d up to 6mo of age. Dairy heifers have been grown at 632g/d or 883g/d from 5d to 6 weeks of age followed by being fed the same diet up until slaughter at 250kg and the calves with higher growth rates were found to have more mammary parenchymal tissue than those with lower growth rates. It was concluded that rapid growth in the calf period had no negative effect on mammary development (Sejrsen, Purup, Martinussen and Vestergaard, 1998).

In some experiments this effect has not been found, which was probably due to short treatment periods, high pre-treatment growth rates, small growth rate differences between treatment groups, variation of growth rates within treatment groups and treatment periods outside the critical periods. However, in a few experiments the absence of treatment effect cannot be explained in this way. This demonstrates that the knowledge on the effect of nutrition during rearing on the future milk yield of heifers was incomplete and that it may be possible to develop high growth rate feeding regimens for heifers. Experimental evidence suggests that the observed negative effects of feeding level on subsequent milk yield are due to impaired mammary development. Development of suitable high growth rate feeding regimens therefore requires understanding of the influence of nutrition on the physiological regulation of mammary development. Data suggest that the growth hormone-insulin-like growth factor I axis was involved, but it was not clear how. It is likely that understanding of the role of insulin-like growth factor binding proteins is important. Alternative hypotheses involve possible effects of growth factors and modifications of mammary tissue sensitivity to hormones and growth factors.

Age, live weight and body condition at first parturition

In dairy heifers there has been found to be an interplay between genetic merit, nutrition and milk yield (Lee, 1997). The dairy heifers with a greater live weight at first calving (Lee, 1997) or a greater percentage of adult weight (Troccon, 1993), have been found to have higher dry matter intakes and greater milk yields during the first lactation. Thus these animals are less susceptible to being unnecessarily culled due to low milk yield. However, despite the importance of weight at first parturition, the liveweight gain of young dairy replacement heifers has been found to have a low heritability and to be a poor indicator of either weight at first calving or first lactation milk yield (Lee, 1997). Fortunately, adult weight has been found to be highly heritable (Lee, 1997) and due to its positive effect on feed intake and milk yield (Troccon, 1993), it provides an excellent indicator of development. As a consequence, the expected adult weight should be used along with age at first calving to develop heifer feeding and management plans, in which these can be used to calculate the growth rates required during heifer rearing to achieve a high level of mature weight at first parturition. Clearly, growth rates and subsequent feeding levels are highly dependent on the desired live weight and age at first calving.

The optimum length of the rearing period i.e. calving age for dairy heifers has typically been approximately 2 years or 24 months of age and the subsequent growth rates required will be dictated by the desired calving live weight. However, data from Dutch dairy heifer rearing has been applied to the development of heifer rearing models. Mourits *et al.* (1999) developed a stochastic (dynamic) model to optimise management decisions with respect to dairy heifer growth rates, insemination and replacement rates. The model maximised the net present value of net returns per heifer place, to achieve economically efficient management decisions. The economic modelling of heifer rearing systems on Dutch and Pennsylvanian dairy farms has found that it was more profitable to rear heifers at the highest achievable growth rates without fattening (Mourits *et al.*, 1999 and 2000 a, b). The optimum practice resulted an average age of first calving of 21.2 months and a body weight of 541 kg on Dutch farms (Mourits at al., 1999) and age at first calving of 20.5 months at a body weight of 563 kg in Pennsylvania (Mourits *et al.*, 2000 a, b). Research and survey data from benchmarking of dairy herds in Northern Ireland indicated that at an average calving age of 24 months Friesian heifers of medium merit were found to have a live weight of 520 kg, while high merit Holstein heifers had a live weight of 600 kg at calving. These age at first calving and live weights were however lower than those stated by NRC (2001) with the calving weight of 641 kg.

The genetic merit and breed of the animal will affect the adult body weight and the body condition score at parturition. Heifers, much like cows which have high levels of body fat (BCS >4.0), at parturition are likely to have dystocia, lower postpartum feed intake levels and a higher incidence of metabolic disorder. In dairy heifers at parturition, adequate body condition has been found to be essential for high milk yield with genetic ability to mobilise body condition to increase milk yield justify higher concentrate feeding levels and resulting in greater total efficiency up to the point of causing digestive disorders (Lee, 1997). This final comment seems a little extreme, but it was clear that heifers require adequate body fat reserves and low body condition were likely to reduce milk yield and poor reproductive performance resulting in increased culling of heifers. A body condition score of 3.0 has been suggested for Holstein dairy heifers (Carson *et al.*, 2003). Clearly genetic merit will play a part in the optimal level of body condition, with high genetic merit having lower body condition in general (2.5 to 3), while body condition of dual-purpose animals such as British Friesian and lower genetic merit animals are likely to be higher (3.5 to 4).

The age at calving was frequently determined by the feed resources available and no two farms are alike in terms of the resources available and the ability to utilise these efficiently (Gabler *et al.*, 2000). Calving age was largely dependent on the feed and land resources available. The economic use of lower quality land resources for heifer rearing may require higher levels of supplementary feeds or dairy cattle to calve above 2 years of age, i.e. 2.5 or 3 years, which was typical on many dairy farms. However, increasing the age at first parturition has the effect of increasing the number of dairy replacements present on the farm at any one time, overall stocking rate of the farm, labour requirements and total heifer rearing costs. The effect of age at first parturition on the number of dairy replacements in differing age levels and stocking rate per 100 cows with a replacement rate of 30 replacements per year are presented in Table 3.

Table 3. The effect of age at first parturition on the number of dairy replacements in differing age levels and stocking rate per 100 cows with a replacement rate of 30 replacements per year

	Age at parturition		
	2	2.5	3
Age groups (months)			
0 to 12	30	30	30
12 to 24	30	30	30
24 to 36	0	15	30
Total number	60	75	90
Stocking rate			
2.0	15.0	21.0	27.0
2.25	13.3	18.7	24.0
2.5	12.0	16.8	21.6

Amended from: Greenmont College

Weight and percentage of adult weight at parturition

Whatever resources available and thus optimal age at first parturition, it was clear that heifers that calve for the first time at a low percentage of adult weight have lower feed intake levels, milk yields and have greater levels of metabolic disorder (Lee, 1997). These animals are more likely to have low yields, poor reproductive performance and be culled from the dairy herd. As a consequence, it would be uneconomic to allow dairy heifers to calve for the first time at a low percentage of adult body weight. In 2001 NRC adopted a post partum live weight of not less than 0.82 of mature body weight for dairy heifers (Van Amburgh, Galton, Bauman, Everett, Fox, Chase and Erb, 1998), while the greatest performance has been found using 0.90 (90%) of inheritable adult live weight at parturition (Van Amburgh *et al*, 1998). Pragmatically the mature size was defined as the herd average for cows in their third or more lactation (NRC, 2001), but the suitability of this approach will depend on the variability within the herd and the rate of genetic change i.e. the breed and breeding policy of the farm. In some situations, i.e. multliple breed use within a herd and rapid change of breed type including within breed and breed changes *per se*, the size of the parents will be a more reliable estimate of mature body weight rather than herd average.

Using the estimated mature body weight, the growth rates required to achieve this can be applied through each of the rearing periods. Thus age and measurements / estimates of live weight should be used together and compared with the target growth rates and live weight for age detailed in a planned management regime throughout the life of the dairy heifer. The addition of these heifer rearing plans to existing farm assurance schemes would help in the internal and external auditing process of assessing and benchmarking of adequacy of nutrition for rearing dairy heifer replacements and work towards increasing the efficiency and profitability of dairy enterprises. To achieve good dairy heifer rearing systems and increase heifer longevity, live weight and growth rate should be measured, documented and compared with the rearing plan at regular intervals, which would be typically achieved at key stages in the development of dairy heifers and cycles of animal management. These include weaning, turn out, housing, live weight at service and as a consequence target live weight at first parturition.

It can however be difficult to obtain accurate weight data in some practical situations and as a consequence other indirect estimates such as bellyband measurement with or without the addition wither height has been used. Condition score here while increasing stature of dairy cattle may be associated with increases in the culling rate and a reduction in the longevity of dairy cattle. In an adequate and nutritionally balanced feeding plan, the live weight of dairy heifers should reflect adequate development, maturity and degree of body fat reserves. Mistakes in the interpretation of live weight into development and maturity could be avoided by using estimates of live weight in combination with body condition score. At parturition, body condition scores of not less than 3.0 and between 3.0. to 3.5 have been recommended for dairy heifers and it would be logical that lower genetic merit dairy cattle and dual purpose animals would have a slightly higher condition score possibly 3.5 to 4.0. However, these are subjective measurements and can be interpreted in a range 0.5 below this by some people when condition scoring animals.

Growth rate and development at service and parturition

The management cycles of dairy heifers typically coincide with the growing season and typically consists of winter housing and summer grazing periods, which provide the opportunity to measure live weight and estimate subsequent development over these periods. In practice, the liveweight gain of young dairy replacement heifers has been found to be highly variable, even over a period of several months (Lee, 1997). This clearly indicates that supplementary feeding levels should not be reduced on a short-term basis. In dairy heifer rearing, the feed plan should be on a long-term basis according to specific live

Figure 3. The live weight according to age of dairy heifer replacement of high calving at 24 (○) 30 (△) and 36 (□) months of age and low genetic merit / dual purpose calving at 24 (●), 30 (▲) and 36 (■) months of age

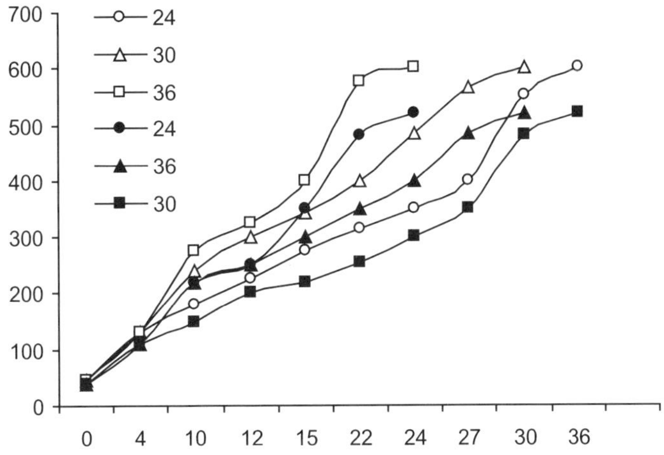

weight targets; the plan should be adhered to and be in sufficient detail to allow internal and external auditing. In particular, supplementary feeding levels should not be altered in the short term in reaction to short term increases in body condition and growth rates. These increases in development rate are likely to be temporary (Lee, 1997) and irregularities in the frequency or level of supplementary feeding will cause inefficient rumen digestion, digestive disorders, reduced growth rate and profitability and would be in contravention of the codes of practice (DEFRA, 2003).

Growth rate and development over the grazing periods

The grazing season was an excellent opportunity to capitalise on the use of forages that have not incurred the cost of preservation. Heifers that graze pasture have been found to have lighter calves at first calving, greater dry matter intakes prior to first calving and during early first lactation than heifers confined indoors, which was likely to be due to greater rumen development and lower condition score at first calving (Troccon, 1993). Moreover, growth and fertility were improved at first lactation (Troccon, 1993). However, while dairy heifers are at pasture, adequate nutrition and levels of supplementary feeding will be dependent on pasture availability, which should be closely monitored by grazing height or other estimates of forage availability. Not surprisingly the greatest growth rates in dairy heifers have been achieved with rotational grazing systems, where grass quality tends to be greater, availability was more easily estimated and parasite infestation can be reduced.

Parasitic infestations of the gastric intestinal tract, lungs and liver are common in dairy heifers. There are a number (18) of parasites of the gastric intestinal tract, however the most common infection in young dairy heifers was *Ostertagiasis ostertagi* infecting the gastric intestinal tract from consumption of pasture previously grazed by infected cattle. This can be minimised by the use of a 'clean' pasture policy or alternatively controlled by the timely use of anthelmintic treatments during the grazing season and during housing to control stage II ostertagiasis developing from L_4 lava. Lung worm (Dictyocaulus viviparus) was also a common parasite affecting young dairy cattle. Growth rates have been found to be greater in calves given a pulse release bolus for the prevention nematode parasitism of lungworm (Talty, McSweeney and Simon, 1996). During the first grazing season, between turnout and housing in mid-July dairy heifers treated for lungworm spend 105 min/d longer grazing, have 0.78 kg dry matter (DM) per day greater herbage intakes and 150 g/d greater daily liveweight gains, compared to non treated herd mates (Forbes *et al.*, 2000). Similarly, irradiated live vaccinations can provide an alternative for the control of moderate levels of lungworm during the first grazing season of dairy heifers. Liver fluke (*Fasciola hepatica*) was an infection gained from the consumption of water from ponds or slow flowing watercourses where the secondary host a water snail (*Lymnaea truncatula*), may be harboured. This disease can be prevented by the fencing off of water sources and wet areas likely to be inhabited by the water snail and allowing access to only piped water from troughs. Alternatively liver fluke can be controlled by the timely use of anthelmintic treatments during the grazing season and at housing or during 'out wintering' where the farm was known to be infected by liver fluke.

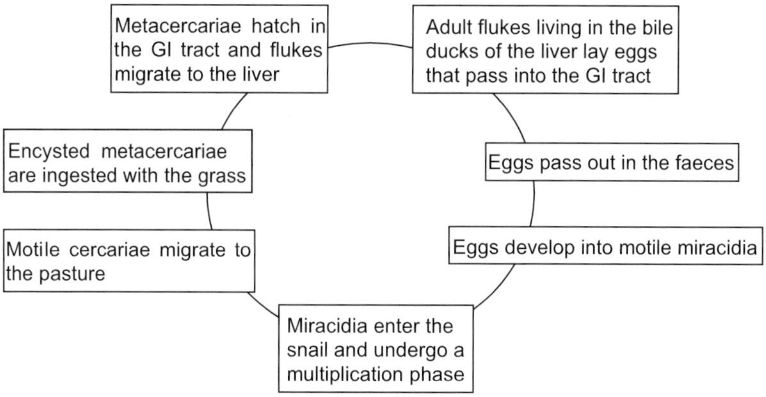

Figure 4. The life cycle of liver fluke (*Faciola hepatica*)

During the grazing season the measurement of live weight can be impractical and as a consequence dairy livestock require frequent visual observation and adequate nutrition levels need to be panned and ensured throughout the season. In any grazing system, the live weight gain during the grazing season could easily be reduced or even live weight gain established can be lost due to periods of parasitism and / or the overestimation of nutritional value of pasture. The lack of pasture availability during the mid grazing season and the overestimation of the feeding value of pasture and parasitism in late summer and autumn are critical periods. In these periods the availability and nutritional value of pasture was frequently overestimated and this can be exasperated by subsequent inadequate supplementary feeding. During grazing periods, the frequent assessment of dairy replacement livestock and forage availability, accurate and realistic estimates of the dietary nutritional contribution of forage, adequate supplementary feeding, timely housing and efficacy of parasite control are important factors in achieving and maintaining liveweight gains and increasing the efficiency of dairy heifer rearing.

Growth rate and development over the winter housing periods

In housing dairy heifers care should be taken to prevent the development of *pneumonia* due to bacterial, viral, mycoplasma, fungal or environmental causes. The causes of possible development of *pneumonia* are presented schematically in Fig. 5. This can be achieved by preventing high levels of environmental load being exerted on housed dairy heifers, by not exceeding recommended building stocking limits, providing good ventilation and avioding mixing or allowing air-space to be shared by heifers from differing age groups. In heifer calf rearing units where viral *pneumonia* can be a particular problem, vaccination against the major causes i.e. RSV and *Pasteurella* by injection and IBR and PI3 by temperature attenuated vaccines are available and should be carried out according to manufacturers' instructions. The parasitic infestation of ostertagiasis during the grazing season can lay dormant in the gastro mucosal glands. This will typically become active and cause a watery diarrhoea and weight loss from February onwards, this stage II ostertagiasis should be prevented by using an anthelmentic treatment at housing.

During housing period, increasing feeding rates and subsequent liveweight gain during consecutive winter feeding periods has been found to increase longevity and milk yield. Troccon (1993) completed an experiment using Holstein dairy heifers, born in the autumn and managed to calve at 2 years of age. In this experiment, an average daily gain (ADG) of 826 and 885 g/d increased the herd life by 333 days, which was also associated with an increased first lactation milk yield by 4089 kg, milk fat yield by 205 kg and milk protein yield 150 kg (Troccon, 1993) compared with heifers with a lower ADG 696 g/d and 639 g/d.

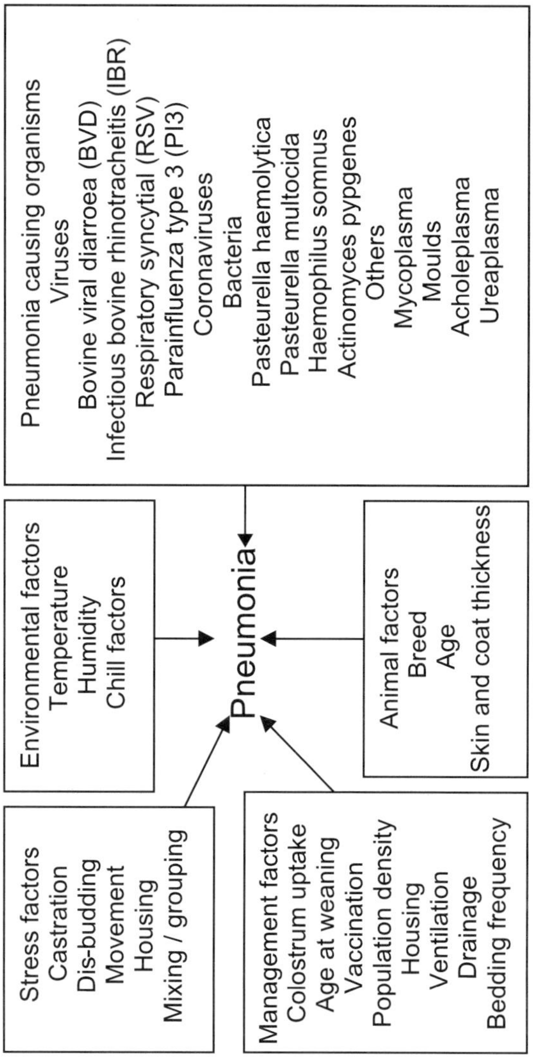

Figure 5. Infectous agents and other factors involved in pneumonia

Growth rate and development

In general high growth rates, without incurring the deposition of fat, have been found to lead to higher milk yields (Troccon, 1993; Van Amburgh *et al*, 1998; NRC, 2001; Sejrsen and Purup, 1997; Knight, 2001). Pre-pubertal growth rates of between 600 to 900 g/d and overall growth rates between 700 to 900 g/d have been used (Troccon, 1993; Van Amburgh *et al*, 1998; NRC, 2001; Segensen and Purup, 1997; Knight, 2001; Carson *et al*., 2003). A proposed target pre-pubertal ADG of 870g (NRC, 2001) has been based on data from beef calves. However, data using even higher rates of growth have been developed using dairy heifers (Troccon, 1993; Van Amburgh *et al*, 1998; Sejrsen and Purup, 1997; Knight, 2001). Higher growth rates are more common in high genetic merit Holsteins, while lower genetic merit and dual purpose animals are reared at lower growth rates. Using data to model the optimum policy in dairy heifer rearing policy, Dutch models were based on a critical prepubertal ADG of 900 g/d and a maximum achievable postpubertal ADG of 700 g/d (Mourits at al., 1999). Moving on to Pennsylvania, Mourits *et al.* (2000) found that a critical prepubertal ADG of 900 g/d and a maximum achievable postpubertal growth rate of 1100 g/d were found to be the optimum practice. The information seems to suggest that high rates of growth can be achieved without reducing milk yield and that higher growth rates increases the milk yield of Holstein dairy heifers. Moreover, the use of sensitivity analysis has found that restrictions on growth rate were found to have a considerable negative effect on optimal rearing practices and the expected net returns (Mourits, 2000). However, in the rearing of all heifers destined to produce milk in the dairy industry it would be important that fat deposition within the developing mammary tissue, particularly during the prepubertal phase, should be avoided (Segensen and Purup, 1997). The growth rates, live weight and percentage of adult weight according to age at parturition and key management stages in the growth and development of dairy heifers are presented in Table 3.

Live weight and development level at service and subsequent parturition

In terms of decision making the level of maturity at service was clearly a watershed in dairy heifers. The live weight at first insemination at 15 months of age has been found to be a better predictor of milk yield than live weight at calving. A target of 0.60 of mature body size at breeding was recommended i.e. 390kg with at mature size of 650kg. The current US guidelines are to inseminate dairy heifers at 0.55 of mature body weight (NRC, 2001). In heifers calving at similar live weights, growth rate during gestation appears to be relatively unimportant (Troccon, 1993; Lacasse, Block, Guilbault and Petitclerc, 1993; Abeni, Calamari, Stefanini and Pirlo, 2000). However, mating at 0.60 of mature weight should allow dairy heifers to calve for the first time at levels approximately 90 % of their inheritable adult live weight (NRC, 2001; Troccon, 1993; Van Amburgh *et al*, 1998) The intentional service of dairy replacements below this level would reduce the milk yield, longevity and profitability of the dairy herd.

As a consequence, dairy heifers should have their development level measured and recorded and animals that have not achieved adequate maturity as indicated by live weight, height and percentage of adult weight (60% of adult weight) should not be served until they have done so. This will enable dairy heifers to achieve their genetic potential, reduce culling rates and efficiency, thus increasing the longevity of dairy cattle and the profitability of dairy herds. The live weight or percentage of adult weight at service was clearly of great importance. However, by regularly monitoring heifer development against a dairy heifer-rearing plan the development can be checked and adjusted prior to service. Should the animals achieve live weights below the targets set out in the management plan then the possibility of increasing feeding levels and growth rates in subsequent phases should be considered. Where this was not or cannot be achieved economically the age at first parturition should be increased. Dairy heifers should calve for the first time at approximately 90 % of adult weight (NRC, 2001) and to achieve this become pregnant at approximately 60 % of adult weight. It would not be either ethical or profitable to intentionally allow dairy heifers to become pregnant or calve below these levels of maturity. To that end, a plan of calving age, target growth rates and live weight should be made. A plan of adequate and appropriate nutrition should be drawn up to achieve these and development should be monitored at regular intervals against these plans. The details of these should be included in the dairy farm assurance standards as part of the responsibility of the management of a dairy herd or dairy heifer-rearing unit. These dairy heifers should also be included in the herd health plan. The successful management of these within the dairy farm assurance standards would increase dairy heifer longevity, productivity and thus farm profits.

Disease and longevity

Lameness

The incidence of lameness in dairy cattle has increased considerably over the past 20 years and according to several surveys (Clarkson *et al.*, 199; Kossaibati *et al.*, 1998) the mean incidence of lameness in individual herds in the United Kingdom varied from 38.2 to 55 cases per 100 cows. Lameness was identified as the third most costly disease of dairy cattle, with mastitis and poor fertility being the most costly (Kossaibaiti and Esslemont, 1997). Lameness has been found to affect the economic performance of dairy cows in several ways: reduced milk yield, loss of body weight, poor fertility, treatment costs and premature culling (Kossaibaiti and Esslemont, 1997; Warnick *et al.*, 2001). Culling due to lameness was 3.5 % in the first lactation and rose to 9 % in the seventh lactation. (Kossaibaiti and Esslemont, 1995). Considering all the direct and indirect costs involved and using data based on 50 herds monitored by the DAISY herd management system,

Kossaibati *et al.* (1999) estimated the cost of lameness for a 100 cow herd to be approximately £4,000 per year, ranging from £1,300 for herds with less lameness problems to £6,800 for herds with a high incidence of lameness. Clearly, reducing the development of lameness and the incidence of mastitis would increase the longevity of dairy cattle and increase the profitability of dairy enterprises.

Housing

In a systematic study of the development of lesions of the claw horn of the sole and white line in heifers calving for the first time, housed either in cubicles or a straw yard and fed either a low or high dry matter forage diet. It was found that both the geometric and cumulative lesion scores increased in all heifer during the first eight weeks postpartum (Webster, 2001). In this research the severity and persistence of the sole and white line lesions were significantly greater in dairy heifers housed in cubicles compared with straw yards. The heels of the cattle in straw yards tended to be thick, but many showed pitting erosions. In contrast, the heels were smooth but thin of heifers housed in cubicles. These differences may have contributed to the development of the claw horn lesions by increasing concessive forces within the hoof (Webster, 2001). The housing of heifers separately from cows during their first lactation and feeding postpartum diets during the prepartum period have been found to increase dry matter intake levels, milk yields and reduce culling rates and extend herd life.

Diet

During early pregnancy feeding Holstein-Friesian heifers higher dry matter diets while housed in cubicles has been found to significantly reduce levels of claw lesion development at 20 weeks *postpartum* (Offer, Leach, Brocklehurst and Logue, 2003; Offer, Fisher, Kempson and Logue, 2001). These experiments measured claw health of Holstein-Friesian heifer calves from three months of age until six months following parturition. Prepartum the heifers were either fed a wet, fermented grass silage-based diet or a dry, unfermented straw and concentrate based diet, apart from grazing during their first summer. Approximately one month prepartum both groups were fed a silage-based diet and following parturition all animals received the same silage and concentrate diet. Claws were examined four times during rearing, once pre-calving, and four times during lactation. In these studies, both white line and sole lesions were significantly greater throughout the first lactation in heifers fed grass silage with less than 25% DM than heifers fed a straw and concentrate diet both during rearing and prepartum. It was concluded that for optimal claw health dairy heifers diets should not be heavily based on wet grass silage with less than 25% DM (Offer *et al.*, 2003; Offer *et al.*, 2001). In a similar study, heifers fed the wet diet had a greater severity of claw horn lesions but this occurred only in the dairy heifers housed the cubicle yard and not in heifers housed in straw yards (Webster, 2001). There were no associations between lesion scores and body weight, body condition or foot conformation. These observations were said to be consistent with the hypothesis that systemic events associated with calving and the onset of lactation may set in motion the chain of events that lead to the development of claw horn lesions. However, the extent and severity of the lesions would then be determined by the externally imposed conditions of housing and feeding (Webster, 2001). This indicates that housing heifers in straw yards during the first lactation would be likely to reduce the severity of sole lesion development and more importantly this has the possibility of reducing the possibility of lameness in their future herd life. However, animals managed in loose housing systems should be frequently bedded with clean dry bedding material (see section on mastitis). The housing of heifers in loose housing can reduce direct culling due to lameness (Webster, 2001; Offer *et al.*, 2001 and 2003). This may reduce culling due to poor milk yield and reproductive performance as a result of reduced dry matter intakes and body condition loss associated with lameness (Margerison *et al.*, 2002). The careful management of heifers during the primiparous period has the possibility of reducing culling and increasing the longevity of the dairy herd, reducing treatment and heifer rearing costs and thus increasing the profitability of dairy enterprises. This would reduce lameness in dairy cattle and the level of economic loss from lameness due to sole lesions and lameness.

Mastitis

At present in the EU and UK, the maximum permitted levels of somatic cell count (SCC) in saleable milk is 400,000 cells/ml. While a reduction in the price paid for milk by milk purchasers can be incurred at levels of SCC above 150,000 cells/ml. As a consequence, reducing the incidence of mastitis and maintaining low milk SCC would be paramount in increasing the longevity of dairy cattle by reducing cull rates and would be central to farm profitability through optimised milk prices and reduced heifer rearing costs. The geometric mean somatic cell count and incidence of mastitis have been found to be higher in dairy cattle loose housed in straw yards compared with those housed in cubicles (MDC, 1998). In addition, SCC has been found to highly correlated and increase significantly (r 0.96, $P<0.005$) with increasing number of lactations completed (Margerison *et al.*, 2000). As a consequence to increase the longevity of dairy cattle, it would be imperative that heifers are prevented where possible from becoming infected with mastitis causing pathogens in order to reduce premature culling due to high SCC. At face value the loose housing of heifers in straw yards may be considered inadvisable and should the system not be well managed this would without a doubt be true. However, closer inspection of data comparing housing systems (Margerison *et al.*, 2000; Macrae, Whitaker, Borrough and Kelly, 2003; Wicks and Leaver, 2003) reveals that the range of SCC in cubicles and straw yards are distinctly different. The range of SCC was consistently greater in cattle loose housed in straw bedded yards and while the highest mean and actual SCC levels were found in this systems so are the lowest SCC levels (Margerison *et al.*, 2000). The lowest SCC in both loose and cubicle housed dairy cattle were highly correlated (r 0.92) with bedding frequency and increased frequency of bedding renewal significantly ($P<0.05$) reduced incidence of mastitis and mean SCC levels (Margerison *et al.*, 2000). Finally, heifers that were habituated to the milking routine have been found to have lower SCC levels. Heifers habituated to the parlour, by passing them through the milking parlour and offering them 1 kg FM of dairy compound for 3 weeks prior to parturition, were found to have significantly ($P<0.001$) lower levels of SCC, higher milk yields and faster milk flow rates compared with heifers introduced to the milking parlour on the day of parturition (Wicks, Carson, McCoy and Mayne, 2003). As a consequence, it was clear that, to ensure the longevity of dairy heifers and reduce culling rates due to SCC levels all points of the 'five point plan' should be applied. In addition particular care should be taken to allow heifers to become accustomed (habituated) to the milking parlour and routine prior to parturition. All dairy cattle should be bedded frequently with clean dry bedding, particularly heifers and those animals housed in loose housing systems, in order to prevent unnecessary infection with mastitis. In addition, heifers could be housed separately from older cows and milked first through the milking parlour to reduce the potential risk of possible infection with mastitis causing pathogens during milking.

In the selection of sires within breeding programmes the opportunity to select sires that have been found to have daughters that have lower levels of mastitis is possible. The selection of sires with increased disease resistance and improved reproductive performance of dairy heifers was an area where the longevity and economic performance of the dairy enterprise can be increased. The restricted nutrition of dairy heifers has been questioned and greater immune levels have been associated with higher feeding levels. In the long term implications of nutrition have been identified. The levels of mastitis in dairy heifers would be no exception and lower levels of mastitis and mortality have been found in heifers fed higher levels of feed during consecutive winter feeding periods (ADG of 826 and 885 g/d). These heifers produced more calves (+0. 9) and had carcass weights 20 kg heavier at culling compared with heifers achieving ADG 696 g/d and 639 g/d during winter feeding periods (Troccon, 1993).

Acknowledgements

Drs J. G. Newbold and K. G. Tanan at the Provimi Research and Technology Centre, Brussels, M. Gold, Volac Ltd, Peterbourough, UK and M. Marsden, ABNA Ltd, Peterbourough, UK, for providing both guidance and information for the preparation of this book chapter.

References

Abeni, F., Calamari, L., Stefanini, L. and Pirlo, G. 2000 Effects of daily gain in pre- and postpubertal replacement dairy heifers on body condition score, bidy size, metabolic profile and future milk production. *Journal of Dairy Science*, 83, 1468-1478.

Arthington, J.D., Cattell, M.B. and Quigley J.D.,III, 2000a Effect of dietary IgG source (colostrum, serum or milk-derived supplement) on the efficiciency of Ig absorption in newborn Hosltein calves. *Journal of Dairy Science*, 83, 1463-1467.

Arthington, J.D., Cattell, M.B., Quigley, J.D., III, McCoy, G.C. and Hurley, W.L. 2000b Passive immunoglobulin transfer in newborn calves fed colostrum or spray-dried serum protein alone or as a supplement to colostrum of varying quality. *Journal of Dairy Science*, 83, 2834-2838.

Bar-Peled, U., Robinson, B., Maltz, E., Tagari, Y., Folman, I., Bruckental, H., Voet, H., Gacitua, H. and Lehrer, A.R. 1997 Increased weight gain and effects on production parameters of Holstein heifer calves that were allowed to suckle from birth to six weeks of age. *Journal of Dairy Science*, 80, 2523-2528.

Baumrucker, C.R., Hadsell, D.L. and Blum, J.W. 1994 Effects of dietary insulin-like growth factor I on growth and insulin-like growth factor receptors in neonatal calf intestine. *Journal of Animal Science*, 72, 428-433.

Brown, M. J. VanderHaar, K. M., Daniels, J. S. Liesman, L. T., Chapin L. T and Weber, M. S. 2002. Increasing energy and protein intake of Holstein heifer calves increases mammary development. *Journal of Animal Science* 80: (Suppl. 1) (Abstr.) 80.

Bühler, C., Hammon, H., Rossi, G.L. and Blum, J.W. 1998 Small intestinal morphology in eight-day-old calves fed colostrum for different durations or only milk replacer and treated with long-R^3-insulin-like growth factor I and growth hormone. *Journal of Animal Science*, 76, 758-765.

Capuco AV, Smith JJ, Waldo DR, Rexroad CE. 1995. Influence of prepubertal dietary regimen on mammary growth of Holstein heifers. Journal of Dairy Science. 78 (12): 2709-2725.

Carson, A. F., Wicks, H. C. F., McCoy, M. A. and C. S. Mayne. 2003. Effects of feeding levels of heifer growth, lactation performance in Holstein Friesian and Danish red cattle. *Proceedings of the British Society of Animal Science, 2003, York, Yorkshire.* 109 - 111.

Clarkson, M. J., Downham, D.Y., Faull, W.B., Hughes, J.W., Manson, F.J., Merritt, J.B., Murray, R. D., Russell, W. B., Sutherst, J. E., Ward, W. R.1996. Incidence and prevalence of lameness in dairy cattle. Veterinary Record. 138 (23): 563-567.

Davenport, D.F., Quigley,J.D., III, Martin, J.E., Holt, J.A. and Arthington J.D. 2000 Addition of casein or whey protein to colostrum or a colostrum supplement product on absorption of IgG in neonatal calves.*Journal of Dairy Science,* 83, 2813-2819.

Davis, C. L. and Drackey, J. K. 1998. The development, nutrition and management of the young calf. Iowa State University Press, Ames, IA. s

Diaz, M. C., Smith J. M. and Van Amburgh, M. E. 1998. Nutrient requirements and management of milk-fed calf. Poceedings Cornell Nutrition Conference, Ithaca, NY. 130-141

Drackley, J. K. 2000. Calf nutrition related to heifer growth and longevity. 61 st. Minisota Nutrition Conference.

Drackley J.K. 2001a Milk feeding strategies for calves does 'accelerated growth' make sense? In *Proceedings of the Professional Dairy Heifer Grower Association* ,National conference, March 22-24, 2001, Seattle, WA.

Durr J. W., Monardes H. G., Cue R. I. and Philpot J. C. 1997. Culling in Quebec Holstein herds. 1. Study of phenotypic trends in herd life. *Canadian Journal of Animal Science.* 77 (4): 593-600.

Forbes, A. B., Huckle, C. A., Gibb, M. J., Rook, A. J., Nuthall, R. 2000. Evaluation of the effects Veterinary Parasitology. 90 (1-2): 111-118.

Gabler M. T, Tozer P. R, Heinrichs A. J. 2000. Development of a cost analysis spreadsheet for calculating the costs to raise a replacement dairy heifer. *Journal of Dairy Science.* 83 (5): 1104-1109.

Gabriel, S, De Bont, J., Phiri, I. K., Masuku, M., Riveau, G., Schacht, A. M., Billiouw M., Vercruysse, J. 2002. The influence of colostrum on early Schistosoma mattheei infections in calves. Parasitology. 125: 537-544.

Girard J. 1986 Gluconeogenesis in late and early neonatal life. *Biology of the Neonate*, 50, 237-258.

Grongnet, J.F., Dos Santos, G.T., Piot, M. and Toullec, R. 1996 Influence of some food additives on IgG plasma concentrations in newborn calves fed an immunoglobulin solution extracted from colostrum. *Lait*, 76, 303-309.

Grongnet, J.F., Dos Santos, G.T., Piot, M. and Toullec, R., 1995 Influence of bovine colostrum thermisation on immunoglobulin intestinal transfer in newborn lambs. *Journal of Animal and Feed Sciences*, 4, 333-339.

Guilloteau, P., Le Huërou-Luron, I.,Chayvialle, J.A., Toullec, R., Zabielski, R. and Blum, J.W. 1997 Gut regulatory peptides in young cattle and sheep. *Journal of Veterinary Medecine*, A44, 1-23.

Hammon, H.M. and Blum J.W. 1997 The somatotropic axis in neonatal calves can be modulated by nutrition, growth hormone and long-R^3-IGF-I. *American Journal of Physiology*, 273 (1), E130-E138.

Hammon, H.M. and Blum, J.W. 1998 Metabolic and endocrine traits of neonatal calves are influenced by feeding colostrum for different durations or only milk replacer. *Journal of Nutrition*, 128, 624-632.

Hammon, H.M., Zanker, I.A. and Blum, J.W. 2000 Delayed colostrum feeding affects IGF-I and insulin plasma concentrations in neonatal calves. *Journal of Dairy Science*, 83, 85-92.

Harp, J.A., Woodmansee, D.B. and Moon H.W. 1989 Effects of colostral antibody on susceptibility of calves to *Cryptosporidium parvum* infection. *American Journal of Veterinary Research*, 50(12), 2117-2119.

Heinrichs, A.J., Well, S.J. and Losinger, W.C. 1995 A study of the use of milk replacers for dairy calves in the United States. *Journal of Dairy Science*, 78, 2831-2837.

Hill, T.M., Aldrich, J/M., Proeschel, A.J. and Schlotterbeck, R.L. 2001 Feeding neonatal calves high levels of milk replacers with different protein and fat levels. *Journal of Dairy Science* 84 (supplement 1), 265 (abstr).

Heinrichs, A.J., Well, S.J. and Losinger, W.C. 1995 A study of the use of milk replacers for dairy calves in the United States. *Journal of Dairy Science*, 78, 2831-2837.

Jagannatha, S, Keown, J. F. and Van Vleck, L. D. 1998. Estimation of relative economic value for herd life of dairy cattle from profile equations. *Journal of Dairy Science*. 81 (6): 1702-1708.

Kertz, A. F., Barton, B. A. and L. A. Reutzel. 1998. Relative efficiencies of wither height and body weight increase from birth until first calving in Holstein cattle. J. Dairy Sci. 81:1479-1482.

Khori, R. H. and F. S. Pickering. 1968. Nutrition of the milk fed calf I. Performance of calves fed on differing levels of while milk relative to body weight. N. N. J. Agric. Res. 11:227-236.

Knight C.H. 2001 Over-fed heifers need not have impaired mammary development. Yearbook 2001: 17. Hannah Research Institute, Ayr, U.K.

Kossaibati, M. A. and R. J. Esslemont. 1997. The costs of production diseases in dairy herds in England. Veterinary Journal. 154 (1): 41-51.

Kossaibati, M. A., Hovi, M. AndR. J. Esslemont. 1998. Incidence of clinical mastitis in dairy herds in England. Veterinary Record. 143 (24): 649-653.

Kossaibati, M. A., Esslemont, R. J. and Watson, C. 1999. The costs of lameness in dairy herds. *Proceedings of the National Cattle Lameness Conference 1999*: (Abst.) 2.

Kühne, S., Hammon, H.M., Bruckmaier, R.M., Morel, C., Zbinden, Y. and Blum, J.W. 2000 Growth performance, metabolic and endocrine traits, and absorptive capacity in neonatal calves fed either colostrum or milk replacer at two levels. *Journal of Animal Science*, 78, 609-620.

Lee, A. J. 1997. The interplay of feeding and genetics on heifer rearing and first lactation milk yield: A review. *Journal of Animal Science*. 75 (3): 846-851.

Le Huërou-Luron, I., Guilloteau, P., Wicker-Planquart, C., Chayvialle, J-A., Burton, J., Mouats, A., Toullec, R.and Puigserver, A. 1992 Gastric and pancreatic enzyme activities and their relathionship with some gut regulatory peptides during postnatal development and weaning in calves. *Journal of Nutrition*, 122,1434-1445.

Levieux, D. and Ollier A. 1999. Bovine immunoglobulin G, lactoglobulin, lactalbumin and serum albumin in colostrum and milk during the early post partum period. *Journal of Dairy Research*, 66, 421-430.

Margerison, J. K., Edwards, R. Randle, H. and Burke, J. 2002. Health and welfare of dairy cattle in organic systems in the South West of England. In: Organic meat and milk from ruminants. Editors: I. Kyriazakis and G. Zervas. Wageningen Academic Publishers. EAAP publication No. 106, 123-126., Athens, Greece. 4-6 October 2001.

Margerison, J. K., Winkler, B. and Stephens, G. 2002. The effect of locomotion score on feed intake and feeding behaviour. Proceedings of the 12th International Symposium on Lameness in Ruminants, 9-12 January 2002, Orlando, USA.

Macrae, A., Whitaker, D., Borrough, L and J. Kelly. 2003. Mastitis trends in UK dairy herds. *Proceedings of the British Mastitis Conference, 2003, Garstang. Lancashire*. 131 –133.

Mee, J. F., O'Farrell, K. J., Reitsma, P. and Mehra, R. 1996 Effect of a whey protein concentrate used as a colostrum substitute or supplement on calf immunity, weight gain and health. *Journal of Dairy Science*, 79, 886-894.

Morin, D. E., McCoy, G. C. and Hurley, W. L. 1997 Effects of quality, quantity, and timing of colostrum feeding and addition of a dried colostrum supplement on immunoglobulin G_1 absorption in Holstein bull calves. *Journal of Dairy Science*, 80, 747-753.

Mourits, M. C. M., Galligan, D, T., Dijkhuizen, A. A., Huirne, R. B. M. 2000. Optimization of dairy heifer management decisions based on production conditions of Pennsylvania. Journal of Dairy Science. 83 (9): 1989-1997.

Mourits, M. C. M., Huirne, R. B. M., Dijkhuizen, A. A. and Galligan, D. T. 1999. Optimal heifer management decisions and the influence of price and production variables. *Livestock Production Science*. 60 (1): 45-58.

Mrode, R.A., Swanson, G. J. T. and Lindberg, C. M. 2000. Genetic correlation's of somatic cell count and conformation traits with herd life in dairy breeds, with an application to national genetic evaluations for herd life in the United Kingdom. *Livestock Production Science*. 65 (1-2): 119-130.

NADIS, National Animal Disease Information Service 1996 UK disease profile - Calf enteritis survey. Report 96/R5/10. Ed. Milk Development Council.

National Research Council. 1989. Nutrient Requirements of Dairy Cattle. National Academy Press, Washington, DC.

Nocek, B. J. and D. G. Braund, 1986. Performance, health and postweaning growth on calves fed cold, acidified milk replacer adlibitum. J Dairy Sci. 69:1871-1883.

Nonnecke, B. J., Van Amburgh, M. E., Foote, M. R., Smith, J. M. and Elsasser, T. H. 2000. Effects of dietary energy and protein on the immunological performance of milk replacer fed Holstein bull calves. Journal of Dairy Science 83 (supp 1) 135 (Abstr.).

Offer, J. E., Leach, K. A., Brocklehurst, S. and Logue, D. N. 2003. Effect of forage type on claw horn lesion development in dairy heifers. Veterinary Journal 165 (3): 221-227.

Offer J, E, Fisher GEJ, Kempson SA, Logue DN. 2001. The effect of feeding grass silage in early pregnancy on claw health during first lactation. *Veterinary Journal*. 161 (2): 186-193.

Owens, F.N., Dubeski, P. and Hanson, C.F. 1993 Factors that alter the growth and development of ruminants. *Journal of Animal Science*, 71, 3138-3150.

Pettersson, K., Svensson, C. and Liberg, P. 2001. Housing, feeding and management of calves and replacement heifers in Swedish dairy herds. *Acta Veterinaria Scandinavica*. 42 (4): 465-478.

Quigley, J.D., III and Drewry, J.J. 1998 Nutrient and Immunity transfer from cow to calf pre- and postcalving. *Journal of Dairy Science*, 81, 2779-2790.

Quigley, J.D., III, Martin, K.R., Dowlen, H.H., Wallis, L.B. and Lamar, K. 1994 Immunoglobulin concentration, specific gravity and nitrogen fraction of colostrum from Jersey cattle. *Journal of Dairy Science*, 77, 264-269.

Quigley, J.D., III, Fike, D. L., Egerton, M.N., Drewry, J.J. and Arthington J.D. 1998 Effects of a colostrum replacement product derived from serum on immunoglobulin G absorption by calves. *Journal of Dairy Science*, 81, 1936-1939.

Quigley, J.D., III, Martin, K. R. and Dowlen H.H. 1995 Concentrations of trypsin inhibitor and immunoglobulins in colostrum of jersey cows. *Journal of Dairy Science*, 78, 1573-1577.

Quigley, J, D. and Wolfe, T. M. 2003. Effects of spray-dried animal plasma in calf milk replacer on health and growth of dairy calves.

Journal of Dairy Science. 86 (2): 586-592.
Radke, B. R., Lloyd, J. W., Tempelman, R. J., Kaneene, J. B., Black, J. R. and Harsh, S. 2000. Parents' predicted transmitting abilities are not associated with culling prior to second lactation of Michigan, USA dairy cows. *Preventive Veterinary Medicine*. 43 (2): 91-102.
Rauprich, A.B.E., Hammon, H.M. and Blum J.W.2000a Effects of feeding colostrum and a formula with nutrient contents as colostrum on metabolic and endocrine traits in neonatal calves. *Biology of the Neonate*, 78, 53-64.
Rauprich, A.B.E., Hammon, H.M.,and Blum J.W. 2000b Influence of feeding different amounts of first colostrum on metabolic, endocrine and health status and on growth performance in neonatal calves. *Journal of Animal Science*, 78, 896-908.
Richard, A. L., Muller, L. D. and A. J. Heimrichs. 1988. Adlibitum or twice daily feeding of acidified milk replacer to calves housed individually in warm and cold environments. J. Dairy Sci. 71:2193-2202.
Royal M. D. Pryce J.E. Wooliams J. A. and Flint A. P. F. 2002. The Genetic Relationship between Commencement of Luteal Activity and Calving Interval, Body Condition Score, Production, and Linear Type Traits in Holstein-Friesian Dairy Cattle. *Journal of Dairy Science* 85: 3071-3080
Royal M. D. Darwash A. O. Flint A.P.F. Webb R. Wooliams J. A. Lamming G. E. 2000, Declining Fertility in dairy cattle: changes in traditional and endocrine parameters of fertility, *Animal Science* 70 487-501.
Sangild, P.T., Fowden, A.L. and Trahair J.F. 2000 How does foetal gastrointestinal tract develop in preparation for enteral nutrition after birth? *Livestock Production Science*, 66,141-150.
Sejrsen K, Purup S. 1997. Influence of prepubertal feeding level on milk yield potential of dairy heifers: A review. Journal of Animal Science. 75 (3): 828-835.
Sejrsen, K. S., Purp, H., Martinussen, H and Vestergaard, M. 1998. Effect of feeding level on mammary growth in calves and prepubertal heifers. *Journal of Dairy Science* 81(Suppl 1):377 (Abstr.).
Schiessler, G., Nussbaum, A., Hammon, H. M., Blum, F. W. 2002.Calves sucking, colostrum and milk from their dams or from an automatic feeding station starting in the neonatal period: metabolic and endocrine traits and growth performance. Animal Science. 74: 431-444.
Smith, J. M., Van Amburgh, A. L. Bork and M. R. Foote. 2000. Response to repeated bST challenge around weaning on Holstin heifet and bull calves. J. Dairy Sci. 83 (Suppl.1):144 (Abstr.).
Steinwidder, A. and Greimel, M. 1999. Economic valuation of longevity of dairy cows. *Bodenkultur*. 50 (4): 235-249.

Talty, P. J., McSweeney, C. and Simon, A. J. 1996. Control of lungworm in dairy calves on a farm in County Clare using doramectin in a treatment programme. Irish Veterinary Journal. 49 (11): 661-663.

Thickett, B., Mitchell, D. and Hallows, B. 1988 Calf Rearing. Second edition. Farming Press, Ipswich.

Tanan, K. G. and J. R. Newbold. 2002. Nutrition of the dairy heifer calf. Nottingham Feed Manufacturers Conference, University of Nottingham - Sutton Bonnington, January 2002.

Tizard, I. R., 2000 Immunity in the fetus and newborn In *Veterinary immunology: an introduction. 6th Edition.*Ed. W.B. Saunders company, Philadelphia. P210-221.

Toullec, R., Lalles, J-P., Grongnet, J-F. and Levieux, D. 2001 Digestion of colostrum by the pre-ruminant calf: digestibility and origin of undigested protein fractions in ileal digesta. *Lait*, 81, 443-454.

Tozer, P. R. 2000. Least-cost ration formulations for Holstein dairy heifers by using linear and stochastic programming. Journal of Dairy Science. 83 (3): 443-451.

Troccon, J. L. 1993. Effects of winter feeding during the rearing period on performance and longevity in dairy-cattle. *Livestock Production Science.* 36 (2): 157-176.

Troccon, J. L. 1993. Dairy heifer rearing with or without grazing. *Annales de Zootechnie* 42 (3): 271-288.

Troccon, J.L. and Toullec, R. 1989 Aliments d'allaitement pour veaux d'élevage. Remplacement de la poudre de lait par d'autres sources protéiques. INRA, *Productions Animales*, 2(2), 117-128.

Van Amburgh, M. E.,Tikofsky, J. N., Tedseschi, L. O., Smith, J. M. and Drackley, J. 2001. Requirements for growth of Holstain calves and evaluation of current feeding systems. Proceedings of Cornell university Conference for Feed Manufacturers, 2001, Ithaca, NY. 46-55.

Van Amburgh, M. E. 2002. Growth and subsequent productivity of dairy replacements. *Journal of Animal Science* 80: (Suppl. 1) (Abstr.) 80.

Van Amburgh, M.E., Galton, D.M., Bauman, D.E., Everett, R.W., Fox, D.G., Chase, L.E. and Erb H.N. 1998 Effects of three pre-pubertal body growth rates in Holstein heifers during first lactation performance. *Journal of Dairy Science*, 81, 527-538.

Van Amburgh, M.E., Tikofsky, J.N., Tedseschi, L.O., Smith, J.M. and Drackley J. 2001 Requirements for growth of Holstein calves and evaluation of current feeding systems. *Proceedings of Cornell Universtity Conference for Feed Manufacturers 2001*, Ithaca, NY. p. 46-55.

VandeHaar M.J. 1997 Dietary protein and mammary development of heifers: analysis from literature data. *Journal of Dairy Science* 80(supplement 1), 216 (abstr).

Webster, A. J. F. 2001. Effects of housing and two forage diets on the development of claw horn lesions in dairy cows at first calving and in first lactation. Veterinary Journal 162 (1): 56-65.

Wicks, H. C. F., Carson, A. F., McCoy, M. A. and C. S. Mayne, 2003. Effects of Habituation to the milking parlour and cow breed on milk flow rates and somatic cell count in early lactation. *Proceedings of the British Mastitis Conference, 2003, Garstang. Lancashire.* 109 -111.

Wicks, H. C. F. and J. D. Leaver. 2003. The influence of housing systems on somatic cell counts. *Proceedings of the British Mastitis Conference, 2003, Garstang. Lancashire.* 105 -107.

Zwald, N. R., Weigel, K, A., Fikse, W. F. and Rekaya, R. 2003. Identification of factors that cause genotype by environment interaction between herds of Holstein cattle in seventeen countries. *Journal of Dairy Science.* 86 (3): 1009-1018.

2

PHYSIOLOGICAL ADAPTATIONS TO MILK PRODUCTION THAT AFFECT THE FERTILITY OF HIGH YIELDING DAIRY COWS

V. J. Taylor[1], D. E. Beever[2] and D. C. Wathes[1]
[1]*Reproduction and Development Group, Royal Veterinary College, University of London, Hertfordshire AL9 7TA, UK;* [2]*Centre for Dairy Research, University of Reading, Berkshire RG6 6AT, UK.*

Summary

The high yielding dairy cow is expected to produce a substantial milk output every year and at the same time to conceive and maintain a pregnancy to term. To fulfil lifetime production potential a balance between yield, fertility and other influential factors has to be achieved. Any inability on the part of the management system to identify and rectify problems or on the part of the cow to cope with metabolic demands invariably results in economic or welfare issues. Our studies of high yielding dairy cows have revealed that some animals are capable of normal reproductive function whilst others are classic repeat breeders (requiring 3+ services per conception) or simply fail to re-breed. It is well established that the somatotrophic axis (growth hormone and insulin-like growth factors) drives lactation in ruminants but it is also intimately involved in reproductive processes. An awareness of metabolic adaptations to lactation that impact on reproduction in dairy cows is needed for appropriate management.

The objective of our studies was to explore the metabolic profiles of high yielding dairy cows to identify factors influencing their ovarian function and fertility, hence to characterise the physiological adaptations involved. Our studies revealed different relationships between progesterone profile categories and metabolic status post partum. Delayed ovulation (DOV) or persistent corpora lutea (PCL) may be an appropriate response to a nutritional state or physiological situation and it may therefore be inaccurate to refer to these as 'abnormal'. Whilst associated with high milk yields, not all profile categories detrimentally affected fertility parameters. Delayed ovulation post-calving (DOV1) was identified as the most prevalent abnormal profile encountered in first lactation high yielding cows. This may have occurred because the cows were not yet physically mature and unable to sustain both milk production and growth. The condition lasted long enough (71 ± 8.3 days from calving) to have a detrimental impact on their overall fertility parameters and was associated with significant physiological changes, representative of tissue mobilisation. Although the incidence of persistent luteal phases (PCL1 and PCL2) in dairy cows is increasing, this condition was not found to have any substantial detrimental effects on fertility or production parameters of the primiparous or multiparous cows in these studies. The main reproductive problems in our high yielding primiparous and multiparous cows appeared to be a failure to ovulate and conceive at the expected time or to maintain a pregnancy. These situations were associated predominantly with high milk yields and low concentrations of plasma IGF-I. A failure to ovulate appears to occur when body reserves are mobilised to maintain milk yield at the expense of reproduction and seems most likely to occur in primiparous high yielding cows or those experiencing GH-resistance (low IGF-I) due to excessive body condition loss, reduced feed intakes and factors such as stress and disease. More detailed investigations of dietary means of increasing IGF-I and optimising insulin concentrations, targeted at important reproductive times, are required in high yielding dairy cows, to aid in their management.

Introduction

High yielding UK dairy cows are routinely producing in excess of 10 000 kg of milk and in the United States up to 14 000 kg per 305 day lactation. In some countries exogenous bovine somatotropin (bST) is also administered to increase yields. There is no clear definition of a high yielding cow as the criteria vary with country, breed and over time, making comparisons between studies difficult. A modern high yielding cow produces notably more milk than a 'high yielding' cow from 10 or 20 years ago. The average yearly milk production of UK Friesian dairy cows was 2500 kg in 1920, 4500 kg in 1980, 5521 kg in 1990 (Lamming, Darwash, Wathes and Ball, 1998) and close to 6500 kg in 1998 in Holstein-Friesians. The milk yield increases achieved over recent decades have provided evidence for an antagonistic relationship between high milk production and reproductive success in dairy cows (Nebel and McGilliard, 1993; Bagnato and Oltenacu, 1994). To achieve an acceptable calving interval, post-calving uterine involution needs to occur without complication for the cow to be receptive for another pregnancy. Dairy cows are generally judged as fertile if they resume reproductive cyclicity following calving before 40 days, are served from about 60 days and conceive close to 80 days *post partum*. Close to the breeding period, the cow reaches her peak milk yield (often in excess of 50 litres per day) and any disturbances to energy or metabolic status at this time are likely to impact on her physical health and affect her ability to conceive.

High yielding animals are of value to the dairy industry and help fulfil consumer requirements as they: maximise profit with fewer animals, enhance production efficiency and nutrient optimisation and reduce environmental concerns as fewer animals produce less waste. Hence lifetime production potential of individual animals increases in both importance and value with increased potential for yield. The dairy industry would benefit considerably from being able to identify at an early age animals unlikely to achieve high milk yields and remain fertile, and from nutritional strategies that ameliorate the detrimental effects of metabolic load on the reproductive status of lactating animals. With improved knowledge it may be possible to manage high yielding animals without compromising their fertility, which would benefit the dairy farmer and improve cow welfare.

Physiological adaptations to increased production represented by individual metabolic characteristics have been investigated, but few clear relationships defining the impact of yield improvement on fertility have emerged. This is partly due to the complicated nature of such interactions. Transitory changes may be hard to detect, whereas paracrine and autocrine effects are difficult to investigate. In addition, many fertility parameters are influenced by other factors such as disease and management decisions. In our studies we have defined ovarian function based on endocrine measures and have investigated the metabolic characteristics associated with different patterns of ovarian function in lactating dairy cows. This paper addresses two linked questions: 1) Is there an unavoidable direct conflict between increased milk yield, ovarian dysfunction and decreased fertility in dairy cows? and 2) Can high milk yield and acceptable fertility be achieved with improved nutrition, management and genetics?

Is there an unavoidable direct conflict between increased milk yield, ovarian dysfunction and decreased fertility in dairy cows?

Physiology of lactation: the somatotrophic axis and increasing milk yields

Growth hormone (GH, somatotrophin) is the major lactogenic hormone in ruminants and increased yield is thought to have been partly achieved by genetic selection for GH. In the early *post partum* period, high yielding animals have higher overall plasma GH (Harrison, Ford, Young, Conley and Freeman, 1990) which promotes lactation, reduced plasma insulin-like growth factor-I (IGF-I) and insulin (Bonczek, Young, Wheaton and Miller, 1988). At the start of lactation many dairy cows are unable to consume enough to meet their energy requirements for maintenance, milk yield and growth and experience a period of negative energy balance

(NEB; Beever, Hattan, Reynolds and Cammell, 2001). NEB can vary in both magnitude and duration. High producing dairy cows mobilise body reserves and lose body condition to maintain their milk production until their intake of feed can match or exceed requirements. This state is further characterised by changes in individual metabolic profiles with, for instance, increases in plasma non-esterified fatty acid (NEFA), betahydroxybutyrate (BHB) and urea levels.

The somatotrophic axis (GH, insulin and IGFs) responds to nutritional changes as well as having numerous effects on the ovarian and uterine systems (see later sections). Many of the somatogenic (proliferative) actions of GH are brought about by plasma IGF-I, which is synthesised and secreted mainly from the liver in response to GH receptor (GH-R) binding. In physiological states of undernutrition, disease or early lactation the relationship between GH and IGF-I uncouples so that IGF-I concentrations do not increase, as expected, despite increases in GH (GH resistance; Thissen *et al.*, 1994; Lang and Frost, 2002). Furthermore, in diseased states, the erosion of lean body mass is a significant factor accounting for increased morbidity and mortality.

Genetics of the GH-IGF-I axis and milk yield

The heritability of milk yield has been estimated as 0.28 (Pryce, Coffey and Simm, 2001) and of GH traits as >0.6 (Sørensen, Grochowska, Holm, Henryon and Løvendahl, 2002). During lactation higher GH concentrations and/or other somatotrophic axis differences result in more available nutrients being partitioned towards the mammary gland instead of other somatic processes. Higher circulating GH concentrations have been reported in lactating dairy animals selectively bred for milk yield (Hart, Flux, Andrews and McNeilly, 1978; Harrison *et al.*, 1990) but as GH is a pulsatile hormone its measurement is complicated. IGF-I concentrations do not fluctuate with feeding activity or diurnally (Ronge, Blum, Clement, Jans, Leuenberger and Binder, 1988) and are a useful clinical marker of nutritional status (Thissen, Ketelslegers and Underwood, 1994).

We monitored average (AGM, mean 305 d yield: 8047 ± 300 kg, n=20) and high (HGM, 305d yield: 10573 ± 245 kg, n=28) yielding multiparous Holstein-Friesian dairy cows with a range of pedigree index (PI) values (+3 to +79). Cows with the lowest PI values tended (P=0.09) to have higher IGF-I concentrations both in the pre-calving and in the early *post partum* period (Figure 1A). In terms of actual milk production, the cows with the lowest 305d yields had significantly (P=0.005) higher IGF-I concentrations and did not show a substantial drop in IGF-I levels after parturition (Figure 1B). Cows with the lowest 305 d yields (5000 to 6000 kg) had significantly (P=0.005) higher IGF-I concentrations post-calving. The 7000 to 8000 kg cows had significantly

(P=0.04) higher IGF-I than the 9000 to 10 000 kg cows. These differences were apparent in the immediate post-calving period, before any quantitative milk yield or dietary intake differences may have had an influence, therefore they are potentially predetermined, developmentally, metabolically and/or genetically.

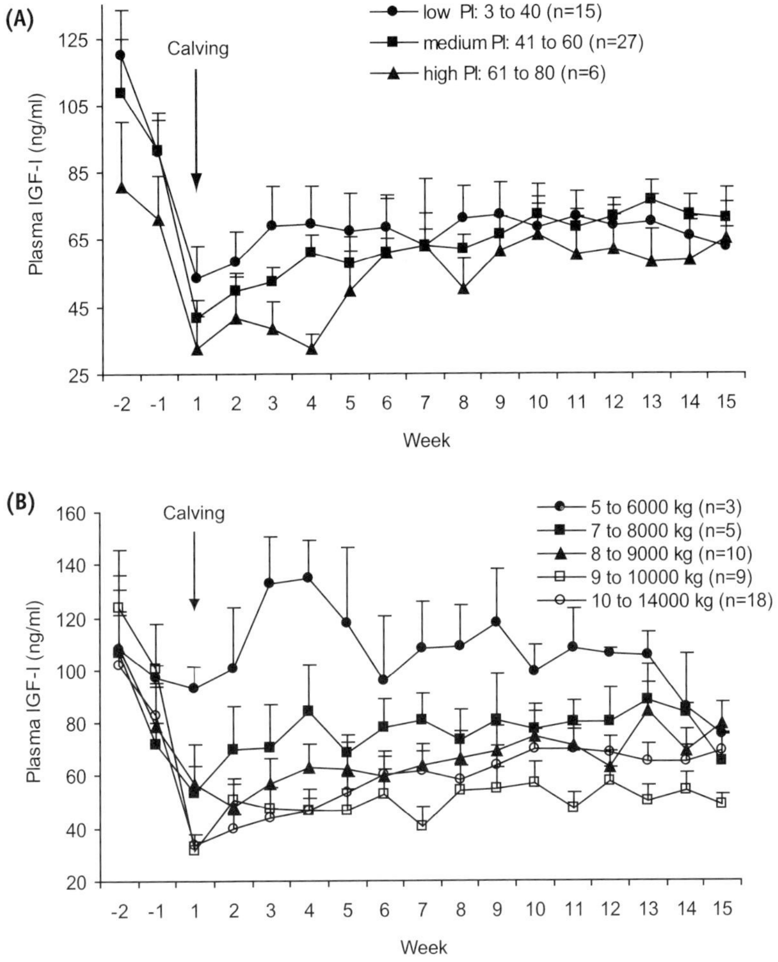

Figure 1. Plasma IGF-I concentrations in average and high yielding cows grouped according to (A) pedigree index (PI) values and (B) 305 day milk yields (mean ± sem).

Several polymorphic regions for the GH gene have been reported in cattle, with two major allelic variants of GH identified and denoted A (leucine) or B (valine) at position 127 (Lucy, Hauser, Eppard, Krivi, Clark, Bauman and Collier, 1993). This polymorphism has been related to milk production traits, although not consistently, and differs between breeds. Grochowska, Sorensen, Zwierzchowski, Snochowski and Lovendahl (2001) found that GH and IGF-I concentrations in response to a thyrotropin-releasing hormone (TRH) challenge were significantly different between young Polish Friesian dairy cattle with different genotypes. The B allele (Val) was favourable for increased GH response whereas the A allele (Leu) was more favourable for IGF-I response. Holstein bulls at 90 and 180 days old had significantly lower IGF-I concentrations than Simmental bulls and these physiological differences were related to GH gene polymorphism (Sirotkin, Chrenek, Makarevich, Huba and Bulla, 2000). GH also increased with age in Holstein cattle but not in Simmentals (Schlee, Graml, Schallenberger, Schams, Rottman, Olbrich-Bludau and Pirchner, 1994). We do not have GH genotypes for the cows studied thus it remains possible that the differences in IGF-I observed could be related to polymorphisms within the group. However, it is clear that with increasing genetic merit and/or milk yields, IGF-I concentrations showed substantial reductions *post partum* in dairy cows.

Genetic influences on fertility

As milk yield has increased there has been a corresponding decrease in the fertility of dairy cows in the UK and US dairy herds (Butler and Smith, 1989; Darwash and Lamming, 1997). Fertility, or infertility, is suspected to have a genetic basis (Pryce, Nielsen, Veerkamp and Simm, 1999) but measures of reproductive performance have low heritabilities (<10%, Hoekstra, van der Lugt, van der Werf and Ouweltjes, 1994; Pryce, Veerkamp, Thompson, Hill and Simm, 1997; Pryce, Esslemont, Thompson, Veerkamp, Kossaibati and Simm, 1998). National dairy selection programmes generally have not included traditional female fertility parameters, partly because they have low or unfavourable heritabilities (Hansen, Freeman and Berger, 1983; Pryce *et al.*, 2001). Scandinavia is an exception and recent studies based there found a reduction in fertility in dairy cows bred only for yield (fertility traits not selected for), when compared with the same breed with fertility traits selected for (Lindhé and Philipsson, 2001). Heritabilities for body condition score (BCS) range from 0.2 to 0.45 and there is a negative genetic correlation between BCS and milk yield (Berry, Buckley, Dillon, Evans, Rath and Veerkamp, 2002). Likewise there is a negative correlation between BCS (adjusted for lactation) with days open of –0.4 (Pryce, Coffey and Brotherstone, 2000) which may be a useful indirect means of selecting for improved fertility.

Lactation is negatively associated with fertility as pregnancy rates in maiden heifers decrease after one or more calvings (Butler and Smith, 1989). We monitored a group of dairy calves from six months of age to the end of their first lactation (mean 305d, 7417 ± 191 kg). Compared with their maiden fertility parameters, there was a decrease in first service conception rates from 54% to 37% and increased number of services required per conception (1.5 ± 0.11 to 2.1 ± 0.24, P =0.04; Taylor, Beever, Bryant and Wathes, 2003). Our higher yielding multiparous animals took significantly longer to resume cyclicity following calving (AGM: 15 ± 1.6 days; HGM: 23 ± 2.3 days; P=0.009). Some published studies are in agreement, for example, Opsomer, Coryn, Deluyker, and de Kruif, (1998) compared their data from modern high yielding herds (mean 305d yield range: 6941 to 9816 kg) with earlier studies and concluded that the first *post partum* ovulation occurred significantly later. This is in contrast to another study where Harrison *et al.* (1990) found that high yield (mean, 10 814 kg) was antagonistic to the expression of oestrous behaviour but not the reactivation of ovarian function, however this was with smaller (n=10 per group) sample sizes. In our study the oestrus detection rate for the second cycle *post partum* was lower in the HGM cows than the AGM cows (32% vs 70%) suggesting that there was also less expression in our high yielding cows. Kinsel, Marsh, Ruegg and Etherington (1998) have recently reported an increase in twinning from 1.4% before 1983 to 2.4% in 1993 concurrent with an increase in milk production. GH is known to positively influence the growth of small follicles and together with lower steroid hormone negative feedback in high yielding animals might increase the probability of twinning. Twinning is especially undesirable in high yielding cows as it adversely affects periparturient health and fertility.

Physiology of *post partum* reproduction

Energy balance, re-establishment of ovarian function and fertility

Ovarian activity and reproductive efficiency following calving are closely related to the cow's energy balance in terms of nutrient intake and milk yield (Butler and Smith, 1989; Lucy, Staples, Michel and Thatcher, 1991). Post-calving, cows resume cyclicity, tend to have a short cycle, followed by at least one full cycle before insemination. Earlier re-establishment of ovarian function is likely to result in more cycles prior to the service period and has been positively associated with improved conception (Thatcher and Wilcox, 1973; Butler and Smith, 1989). The *post partum* onset of reproductive cycles occurs in the NEB period (Senatore, Butler and Oltenacu, 1996) but past its nadir. Our HGM cows were estimated to have a greater negative energy balance (NEB) both in magnitude and duration, with AGM animals achieving positive EB initially at week 6 compared with HGM animals at week 16 (Figure 2; Beever *et al.*, 2001).

Normal and abnormal patterns of ovarian activity

The two main types of abnormal ovarian function identified by milk progesterone analysis are delayed ovulation (DOV) or persistent corpus luteum (PCL). Delayed ovulation describes either a delay in the resumption of ovarian activity post-calving (<45 days) or the development of ovarian cysts either immediately post-calving or following the establishment of progesterone cycles (low progesterone >12 d). Persistent luteal function describes an extended luteal phase (>19 d). It is thought to be due to a failure of the luteolytic mechanism which may be accompanied by uterine infection. Relatively little is known about the specific mechanisms that cause abnormal or atypical progesterone profiles in the pre-service *post partum* period in dairy cows; possible causes have recently been reviewed (Wathes, Taylor, Cheng and Mann, 2003).

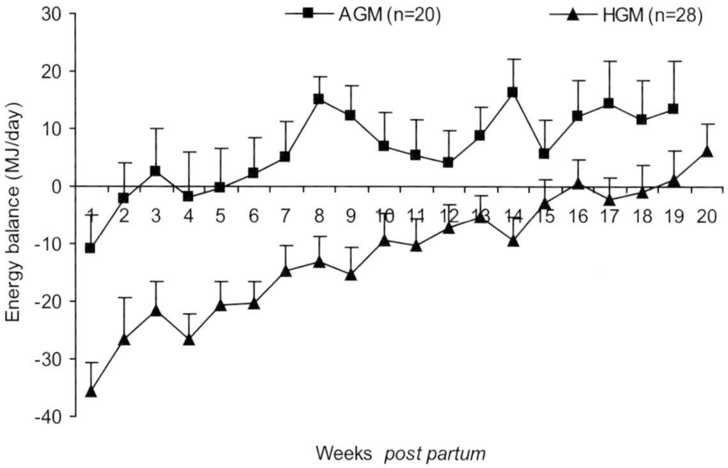

Figure 2. Energy balance (EB in MJ ME/day) for AGM (weeks 2 to 20) and HGM (weeks 1 to 20) cows (mean ± sem).

Reproductive performance in high yielding dairy cows is often less than optimal, with relatively high incidences of ovarian dysfunction (see Table 1) and poor conception rates. Bulman and Wood (1980) documented the incidence of progesterone profile categories in 583 dairy cows (3 Friesian and 1 Ayrshire herd) and found that 12% had abnormal profiles (Table 1). Lamming and Darwash (1998) showed that 32% (794/2503) of profiles monitored between 1975 and 1982 (including data from Bulman and Wood, 1980) had one or more atypical patterns. Royal, Darwash, Flint, Webb, Woolliams and Lamming (2000) found that this had increased to 44% (312/714) in animals studied between 1995 and 1998 and it is notable that a significant increase in the incidence of persistent luteal phases in dairy cows has occurred over the past 25 years (Lamming and Royal, 2001). In Belgian high yielding herds, 47% of cows had abnormal profiles (Opsomer *et al.*, 1998). Our multiparous Holstein-Friesian higher yielding dairy cows experienced significantly (χ^2, P=0.045) more abnormal progesterone profiles (AGM: 30%; HGM: 61%) in the *post partum* period (Taylor Hattan, Bleach, Beever and Wathes, 2001). Further trials with HGM cows (n=56) produced similar results, with approximately 60% abnormal profiles (305d yields: 9475 ± 250, Taylor, Beever, Wathes, unpublished observations).

Lamming and Darwash (1998) found that cows with abnormal progesterone profiles had significantly poorer fertility parameters than those with normal profiles (delayed conception, more services per conception, reduced first service rates and reduced total conceptions). Royal *et al.* (2000) found that cows with abnormal cycles had reduced first service rates, the magnitude of which depended on the abnormal profile category. A delayed resumption of ovulation (DOV1) and the occurrence of a persistent corpus luteum (PCL1) in the immediate post-calving period particularly affected our higher yielding multiparous cows. The multiparous HGM animals with persistent luteal phases (PCL1 and PCL2) and those which had ceased to cycle (DOV2) tended to have more services per conception and took longer to conceive. The DOV2 category appeared to have the most detrimental effect on HGM reproductive parameters in this study. Most of the high yielding multiparous cows in our studies were cyclic by the service period hence their reproductive problems were in establishing or maintaining a pregnancy. Fifty-five percent of our first lactation cows were classified as having abnormal profiles and in this age group, DOV1 (24%) was the most prevalent abnormal profile that lasted for a mean of 71 ± 8.3 days. The DOV1 profile had an adverse effect on subsequent fertility parameters, increasing the number of services required per conception and days open. The primiparous cows with delayed ovulation therefore had not generally resumed cyclicity by the service period. In contrast the PCL1 cows had similar fertility parameters to normal profile primiparous cows. Age of the animal and timing of abnormal progesterone profiles *post partum* therefore influenced the effects on fertility parameters in our high yielding dairy cows.

The energy balance of high yielding cows was found to be correlated with the quality of oocytes (Kendrick, Bailey, Garst, Pryor, Ahmadzadeh, Akers, Eyestone, Pearson and Gwazdauskas, 1999). In a recent study, Snijders, Dillon, O'Callaghan and Boland (2000) demonstrated that the genetic merit of cows (not actual yield) affected oocyte quality; oocytes from HGM cows also resulted in fewer blastocysts produced. These results both support the suggestion that poorer quality oocytes probably also contribute to the reduced conception rates seen in HGM cows. Another notable characteristic of our HGM cows was the number that failed to conceive despite repeated AI attempts (eg HGM vs AGM, 82% vs 100% conceived).

Ovarian function and milk yields

HGM multiparous cows had significantly ($P<0.001$) higher milk yields than AGM cows throughout the study period. Mean peak yields were 52 ± 1.2 kg/day and 37 ± 1.2 kg/day respectively at week 6 ($P<0.001$, t-test). AGM cows with abnormal progesterone profiles produced significantly ($P<0.03$) less milk from week 6 of lactation (after peak yield) than those with normal ovarian function. Conversely, HGM animals with abnormal profiles produced significantly more milk both

Table 1. A comparison of the incidence of normal and abnormal progesterone profiles in dairy cows from different studies (H-F=Holstein-Friesian; DOV=delayed ovulation; PCL=persistent corpus luteum; 1=first cycle *post partum*; 2=later cycles).

	UK Friesian and Ayrshire[#] *1975-78*	*UK Friesian*[†] *1975-82*	*UK H-F*[‡] *1995-98*	*UK difference*	*Belgian H-F*[§] *1990-94*	*AGM***	*HGM***	*First lactation***
Normal	78%	68%	56%		54%	70%	39%	45%
DOV1	5%	11%	13%	~	21%	0%	11%	24%
DOV2	5%	13%	11%	~	3%	10%	18%	4%
PCL1	} 2%	7%	18%	↑11%	} 20%	15%	21%	16%
PCL2		6%	17%	↑11%		5%	11%	11%
Total ABNORMAL	12%	32%*	44%	↑12%	47%	30%	61%	55%

[#]Bulman and Wood (1980); [†]Lamming and Darwash (1998); [‡]Royal *et al.* (2000); [§]Opsomer *et al.* (1998); **RVC/CEDAR studies
*includes some animals with 2+ abnormal profiles; there were minor differences between studies in the definitions of the profile classifications.

at the peak of their lactation curve ($P<0.001$; Figure 3) and throughout their 305d lactation period ($P<0.01$). These data suggest that for high yielders producing >45 kg/d peak yields, milk yield may be related to the incidence of ovarian disturbances. The opposite trend in the AGM cows may suggest that other factors such as disease may have had an adverse influence on both milk production and ovarian function.

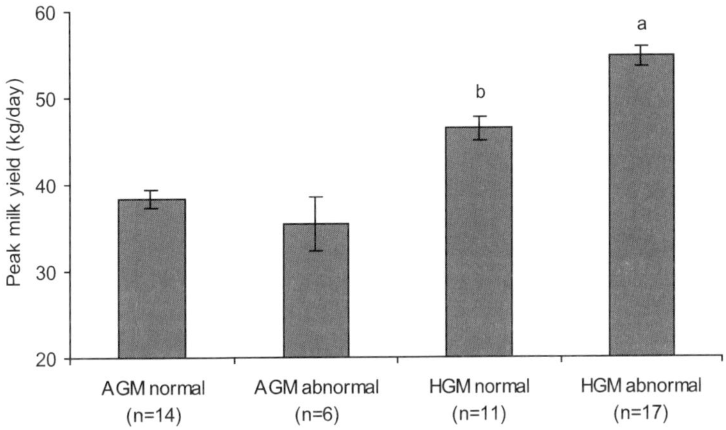

Figure 3. Average daily peak milk yields (mean ± sem in kg/day) for AGM and HGM cows with normal or abnormal progesterone profiles (a>b, $P<0.001$).

All HGM cows with abnormal profiles had significantly ($P<0.01$) higher peak milk yields than those with normal cycles (Figure 4). However, only the delayed start animals (DOV1) had similar 305 day lactation yields to normally cycling animals, whilst the other three abnormal categories had significantly ($P=0.02$; Figure 4) higher 305d milk yields. Presumably the multiparous DOV1 cows were experiencing increased metabolic stress during early lactation and partitioned nutrients away from the reproductive tract to sustain milk production but could not maintain this situation throughout their entire lactation. These relationships between high milk yield and ovarian function were not observed in primiparous or AGM multiparous cows. The first lactation cows were still growing and likely to be under other nutrient partitioning constraints. These data suggest that the relationship between milk yield and fertility is influenced by age and individual metabolic responses to yield and that these aspects of nutrient partitioning contribute towards observed fertility status.

Can high milk yield and acceptable fertility be achieved with improved nutrition, management and genetics?

Our studies of high yielding dairy cows have revealed that some animals are capable of normal reproductive function whilst others are classic repeat breeders (requiring 3+ services per conception) or simply fail to

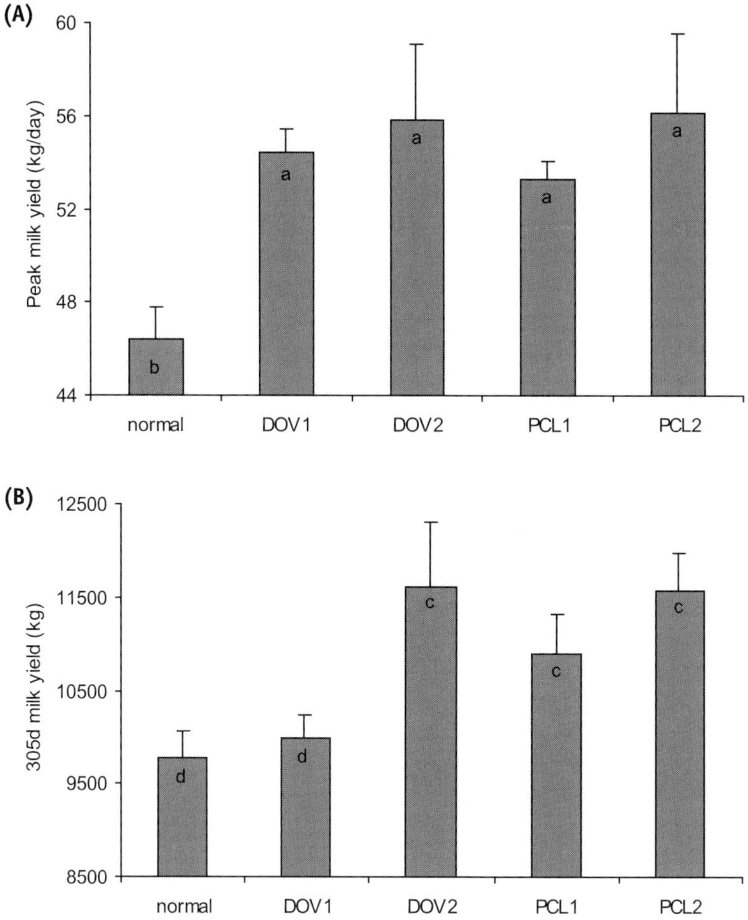

Figure 4. (A) Peak and (B) 305 day milk yields for HGM cows with normal and abnormal progesterone profiles (mean ± sem; a>b, $P<0.01$; c>d, $P<0.05$).

conceive (normal vs repeat breeders vs not pregnant, 51% (25/49) vs 31% (15/49) vs 18% (9/49), Taylor, Beever, Wathes, unpublished). It is important to determine how some cows manage to produce high milk yields and at the same time conceive and maintain their pregnancies whilst others cannot achieve these simultaneously. The differences are possibly due to how various components of the somatotrophic axis influence the reproductive compartments within individual animals. If animals with attributes for fertility and yield can be identified and selected for, it may then be possible to produce animals suitable for current management systems.

The somatotrophic axis and nutrition: physiological responses

Postnatal growth in mammals is regulated by the somatotrophic axis (Gatford, Egan, Clarke and Owens, 1998) although GH, insulin and IGF-I have numerous other important functions and metabolic effects which persist beyond the major growth phases, affecting protein, carbohydrate and fat metabolism. GH stimulates productive processes including growth and cellular survival, reproduction and milk synthesis and promotes homeorhetic adaptations to provide nutrients for these actions (Bauman and Currie, 1980; Etherton and Bauman, 1998). GH has direct effects on cell growth and differentiation, but many of its growth-promoting actions are via stimulation of IGF-I synthesis and secretion, notably from the liver (the 'somatomedin hypothesis'; Figure 5A). The pulsatile pattern of GH release is affected by several factors including feeding, activity, sleep and stress. The classic model of GH pulsatility proposes that it is driven mainly by GRF secretion and modulated by somatostatin release. Low basal GH release is controlled positively by GRF and negatively by somatostatin whereas sex steroid hormones (eg oestradiol) and normal puberty attainment augment GH secretory bursts 1.8 to 3.5 fold (Veldhuis, Anderson, Shah, Bray, Vick, Gentili, Mulligan, Johnson, Weltman, Evans and Iranmanesh, 2001).

(A)

(B)

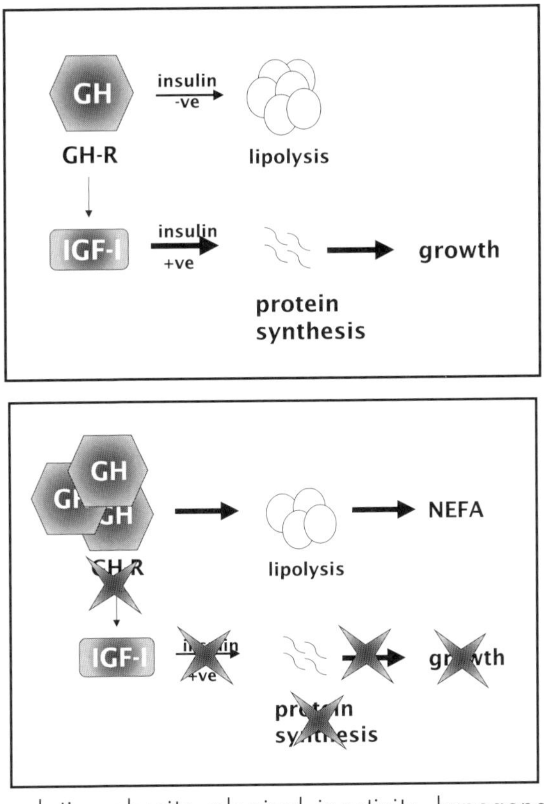

Figure 5. Schematic representations of (A) the normal GH-IGF-I axis and (B) the GH-resistant state.

Aging, relative obesity, physical inactivity, hypogonadism and hypothyroidism blunt the amplitude and mass of pulsatile GH output. Systemic IGF-I changes slowly and damps GH pulse amplitude by delayed negative feedback in an autoregulatory loop. The GH axis is under a complex regulatory system and GH secretion can be precisely regulated under diverse physiological circumstances (Gracia-Navarro, Castano, Malagon, Sanchez-Hormigo, Luque, Hickey, Peinado, Delgado and Martinez-Fuentes, 2002).

Metabolic effects and nutritional regulation of the somatotrophic axis

The somatotrophic axis responds to nutritional changes. Insulin-induced effects are acute and reversible, an adaptation presumably evolved due to episodic feeding and hence likely to be important for rapid metabolic regulation (Ronge *et al.*, 1988). IGF-I concentrations do not fluctuate with feeding activity or diurnally (Ronge *et al.*, 1988). IGF-I acts as a co-factor and optimal concentrations are required, especially for GH to produce maximal effects in normal physiological situations. There may be a critical threshold of nutrient deficit before IGF-I decreases (Thissen *et al.*, 1994). Physiological 'insults', such as nutritional stress, or injury, activate the hypothalamic-pituitary axis (HPA) and elevated circulating glucocorticoids lead to GH resistance (Figure 5B; Clark, 1997). High GH with low IGF-I and insulin concentrations is an endocrine situation that favours lipolysis (in combination with a reduction of triglyceride accumulation via inhibition of lipoprotein lipase, Nam and Lobie, 2000), making free fatty acids available during undernourishment (Figure 5B; Dominici and Turyn, 2002). Fasting results in substrate-sparing metabolic changes: increased production and use of ketone bodies, changes in insulin sensitivity and reductions in glucose use by peripheral tissues; all of which minimise glucose use, and spare amino acids and tissue proteins. This hormonal system probably evolved to cope with inevitable periods without food. Ronge *et al.* (1988) demonstrated that levels of energy were more important than protein in influencing the *post partum* concentrations of IGF-I and insulin in dairy cows. However the energy and protein balances of the cows were strongly correlated, making it impossible to separate their individual effects. Interactions in the rumen make it more difficult to demonstrate specific effects of energy or protein on IGF-I concentrations compared with non-ruminant animals (McGuire, Vicini, Bauman and Veenhuizen, 1992). Circulating insulin concentrations are a stimulus for IGF-I production (McGuire, Dywer, Harrell and Bauman, 1995) but are reduced when dietary protein is restricted (Fliesen, 1989). Of particular note is recent *in vitro* work that found methionine to be the key limiting amino acid involved in the modulation of IGF-I expression in the ovine liver (Stubbs, Wheelhouse, Lomax and Hazlerigg, 2002). Actions resulting from IGF-I stimulation, ie mitosis or differentiation, require anything from six hours to several days to complete (McCusker, 1998). Thus IGF-I concentrations must be maintained for such events to be completed. This is partly achieved by the six binding proteins (IGFBPs 1 to 6) that help to maintain a pool of circulating IGF (Hossner, McCusker and Dodson, 1997). Therefore the IGF-I system can potentially influence events from days to weeks in advance. IGFBPs provide a buffer against decreased IGF-I but not indefinitely. Hence non-essential processes will be restricted until conditions improve and IGF-I concentrations recover. GH/IGF resistance suppresses anabolism in the short-term but chronic suppression ultimately leads to bone marrow depletion and compromised immune function.

Plasma insulin-like growth factor-I (IGF-I) concentrations were consistently higher in lower yielding AGM cows compared with higher yielding HGM cows ($P<0.001$) and increased gradually following calving (Figure 6A). We have previously shown that IGF-I concentrations are higher in primiparous compared with multiparous lactating dairy cows (Wathes, Beever, Cheng, Pushpakumara and Taylor, 2001). The AGM cows also had significantly ($P=0.04$) higher insulin levels than the HGM cows during early lactation (Figure 6B).

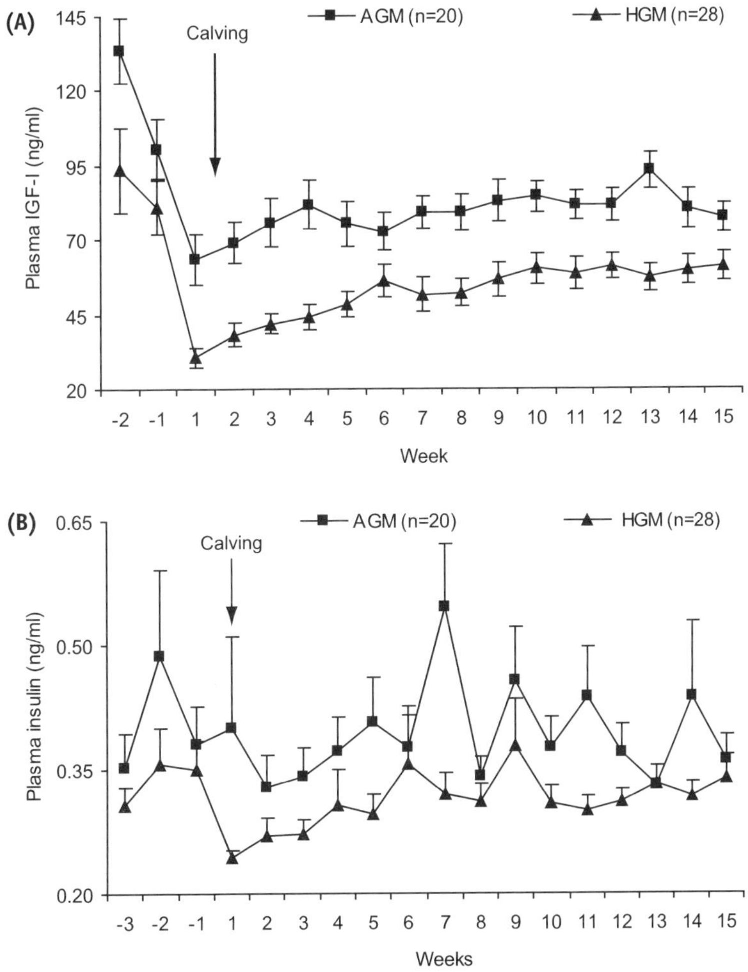

Figure 6. Plasma (A) IGF-I and (B) insulin concentrations in AGM (n=20) and HGM cows (n=28) from pre-calving to 15 weeks *post partum* (mean ± sem).

Over and under expression of GH, IGF-I and insulin

GH and IGF-I are potent anabolic hormones that increase cellular metabolism (increasing glucose use and oxygen uptake) and enhance the function of numerous tissues, especially during development when concentrations are high. When bST is administered to dairy cows during positive EB, GH, insulin and IGF-I concentrations increase. There are a number of human conditions and mice experimental models with alterations of the GH-IGF axis. Growth hormone insensitivity (GHI) is characterised by elevated GH with IGF-I and IGFBP-3 deficiency (eg Laron syndrome, Savage, Burren, Blair, Woods, Metherell, Clark and Camacho-Hubner, 2001). Genetic defects can cause hypothalamic or pituitary GH or IGF-I deficiency (Parks, 2001) and alterations in the somatotrophic axis are found in intrauterine growth restricted (IUGR) offspring and diabetics. Over-expression of GH affects nutrient partitioning and resulted in decreased insulin receptors (IR), IR substrate-1, IR substrate-2 tyrosyl phosphorylation in response to insulin in skeletal muscle and chronic overactivation of the IR substrate-P1 3-kinase pathway in the liver (Dominici and Turyn, 2002). Transgenic mice gained weight faster whilst consuming the same or less food per gram body-weight than normal animals; they slept more and had reduced activity. A disproportionate amount of their metabolisable energy (ME) was used for growth and less for maintenance and reproduction. Their estimated energy deficits were suggested to be responsible for their reduced reproductive performance and reduced lifespans as sucrose supplementation improved both (reviewed by Bartke, Chandrashekar, Turyn, Steger, Debeljuk, Winters, Mattison, Danilovich, Croson, Wernsing and Kopchick, 1999). This 'energy stress paradigm' suggests that excess GH effects on fertility and aging may be due to GH effects on food intake, growth rate and allocation of energy reserves rather than to altered release of hypothalamic, pituitary or adrenal hormones.

The natural ligand for the growth hormone secretagogue receptor (GHS-R), ghrelin, has been discovered in the stomach (Kojima, Hosoda, Matsuo and Kangawa, 2001) and recent work has implicated ghrelin in the regulation of food intake, body weight and energy homeostasis. Hayashida Murakami, Mogi, Nishihara, Nakazato, Mondal, Horii, Kojima, Kangawa and Murakami (2001) found that plasma ghrelin concentrations in cows decreased significantly one hour post-feeding, before recovering. Ghrelin may be involved in the regulation of GH secretion, especially in relation to feeding and it would be useful to explore ghrelin profiles in dairy cows from different genetic lines and with different feed intakes. GH deficient transgenic mice live longer than wild-type controls. Transgenics with high GH exhibit depressed hepatic catalase (an antioxidative enzyme), have increased oxidative damage to tissues and shortened (halved) lifespans. GH and IGF-I may suppress antioxidative enzyme activity *in vivo*. Increased metabolism in association with elevated GH or exogenous GH treatment could increase the production of free radicals (Brown-Borg Rakoczy, Romanick and Kennedy, 2002). Further aging effects associated with GH that have been observed include reduced replicative potential of cells *in vitro*.

Somatotrophic axis and reproduction: ovary and corpus luteum

Endogenous IGF-I concentrations peak at puberty and GH and IGF-I decrease gradually thereafter. GH is directly involved in ovarian regulation via the GH-R, as well as initiating effects via the IGF system systemically and locally (Chase, Kirby, Hammond, Olson and Lucy, 1998), including folliculogenesis (Eisenhauer, Chun, Billig and Hsueh, 1995; with and without FSH, reviewed by Childs, 2000), ovulation rate (Danilovich, Bartke and Winters, 2000), steroidogenesis and lactation. The mechanisms by which GH achieves these effects are only beginning to be unravelled. There is also evidence that GH acts as a co-gonadotroph (Childs, 2000). There are GH-R in granulosa cells of different sized follicles (Kölle, Sinowatz, Boie and Lincoln, 1998a). GH is also involved in the formation and differentiation of granulosa lutein cells (Kölle *et al.*, 1998a). GH-R 1B mRNA has been localised in adult bovine corpus luteum (CL) (Lucy, Boyd, Koenigsfeld and Okamura, 1998) and GH has a direct action by stimulating progesterone and LH-R production (Kirby, Thatcher, Collier, Simmen and Lucy, 1996). The IGF system is active in the female bovine reproductive tract throughout the oestrous cycle and pregnancy (Kirby *et al.*, 1996; Robinson, Mann, Gadd, Lamming and Wathes, 2000). *In vitro* work has demonstrated that IGFs influence the effects of gonadotropins on growth and differentiation. In ovarian tissues of numerous species, IGF-I stimulates granulosa and luteal cell mitogenesis *in vitro* and amplifies gonadotrophin action in granulosa and thecal cells. IGF-I also promotes oestradiol synthesis and aromatase mRNA expression (Hammond, Mondschein, Samaras, Smith and Hagen, 1991; Wathes, Perks, Davis and Denning-Kendall, 1995; Perks, Peters and Wathes, 1999). FSH positively enhances IGF-1R levels so it would seem that both hormones exert a positive feedback loop on each other's receptors (Minegishi, Hirakawa, Kishi, Abe, Abe, Mizutani and Miyamoto, 2000). Granulosa cells are a site of IGF-I (in humans, pigs, rats and mice but not in cows, Perks *et al.*, 1999) and IGFBP production (Davoren and Hsueh, 1986; Wandji, Gadsby, Simmen, Barber and Hammond, 2000), reception and action (Spicer, Alpizar and Echternkamp, 1993; Hugues, Miro, Smyth and Hillier, 1996; Schoppee, Armstrong, Harvey, Whitacre, Felix and Campbell, 1996). Follicular fluid contains many growth factors, including IGF ligands and BPs. As the majority of follicular fluid IGF-I in ruminants is derived from the circulation (Leeuwenberg, Hudson, Moore, Hurst and McNatty, 1996), the availability of IGF-I to follicles is likely to be reduced when plasma levels are low. However less *in vivo* work has been done thus it is unresolved to what extent intra or extra ovarian sources of IGF-I contribute to ovarian functions. Schoppee *et al.* (1996) provided the first evidence that chronic nutrient restriction decreased bovine follicular fluid IGF-I and that the most affected follicles were those not yet selected, hence FSH was unable to support normal follicular function in the absence of sufficient IGF-I.

The bovine CL is a site of IGF-I mRNA expression, peptide production and action (Einspanier, Miyamoto, Schams, Muller and Brem, 1990; Perks *et al.*, 1999). *In vitro* studies in heifer CL tissue by Sauerwein, Miyamoto, Gunther, Meyer and Schams (1992) using a microdialysis system found that insulin and IGF-I (unbound) stimulated the release of progesterone, with IGF-I being the most effective. IGF-I continued to stimulate progesterone secretion after the time of peptide infusion. The greatest stimulation occurred in the late luteal phase (days 15 to 18) when basal progesterone was lowest and suggests that IGF-I may be important at this time to maintain CL function. Insulin stimulated cell proliferation, enhanced FSH-induced oestradiol production *in vitro* (Spicer and Echternkamp, 1995) and progesterone production (Staples, Burke and Thatcher, 1998). Studies inducing diabetes indicate that reduced insulin secretion detrimentally affects oocyte fertilisation in mice as they had a lower percentage of zygotes and an increased percentage of unfertilised and degenerate oocytes compared with control animals (Vesela Cikos, S., Hlinka, D., Rehak, P., Baran, V.and Koppel, 1995).

Work with an animal model - GH receptor deficiency cattle - with similar physiological responses to the undernourished state, has also demonstrated the importance of GH, GH-R and IGF-I to the normal functioning of follicular dynamics and CL development (Chase *et al.*, 1998). Active immunisation of heifers and sows (Armstrong, Harvey, Heimer and Campbell, 1993; Armstrong, Coffey, Esbenshade, Campbell and Heimer, 1994) against GRF decreased IGF-I concentrations, delayed puberty and decreased follicular development and the number of DFs. The later stages of follicular development are influenced by energy restriction with DFs reducing in size and number (Murphy, Enright, Crowe, McConnell, Spicer, Boland and Roche, 1991; Mackey, Sreenan, Roche and Diskin, 1999). Substantial evidence is also available that reduced or excessive GH concentrations can influence reproductive functions (reviewed by Bartke *et al.*, 1999). Animals administered bST and transgenics overexpressing GH have an increased number of small follicles (reviewed by Bartke *et al.*, 1999) and bST has been associated with an increased twinning rate in cattle (Esteban, Kass, Weaver, Rowe, Holmberg, Franti and Troutt, 1994).

Alterations in the somatotrophic axis as a result of selection for milk yield in combination with nutritional adjustments to metabolic load in high yielding dairy cows clearly have the potential to influence all levels of the mammalian reproductive axis, from gonadotrophin release to oocyte quality and embryo survival. Our studies have characterised and revealed metabolic adaptations that result in distinct ovarian conditions, namely delayed ovulation (DOV) and persistent CL (PCL) progesterone profiles (see next section). Why particular animals develop these conditions may be due to transitory endocrine changes but we have some evidence to suggest that certain animals may have predispositions to certain profiles depending on their endogenous hormone concentrations (Taylor, Bryant, Beever and Wathes, unpublished).

The uterine environment, establishment of pregnancy and embryonic development

The GH-IGF system has important roles in the maintenance of the reproductive tract and survival of the embryo. Failure to conceive is the main reason for culling dairy cows (31%, Nielson, Veerkamp, Pryce, Simm and Oldham, 1997). Robinson *et al.* (2000) showed that IGF-I mRNA expression was highest at oestrus in the luminal epithelium of the uterus. Uterine glandular secretions sustain pre-implantation conceptuses. Early embryos (day 13) have GH-R and IGF-1R mRNA as do multiple locations in the reproductive tract (Kölle, Sinowatz, Boie, Lincoln and Waters, 1997; Kölle, Sinowatz, Boie, Lincoln, Palma, Stojkovic and Wolf, 1998b; Robinson *et al.*, 2000; Pushpakumara, Robinson, Demmers, Mann, Sinclair, Webb and Wathes, 2002). Early embryo loss due to failure of maternal recognition of pregnancy is thought to account for 25% of conception failures in dairy cows (Sreenan and Diskin, 1983). Kirby *et al.* (1996) found that lactating dairy cows that conceived had the highest IGF-I mRNA expression. The IGF ligands have important roles regulating the growth of embryonic and extraembryonic tissues during pregnancy. The expression of mRNAs for IGFBPs 1, 2 and 3 were influenced by the presence of an embryo in the ruminant reproductive tract (Osgerby, Gadd and Wathes, 1999; Robinson *et al.*, 2000) and may regulate IGF actions there.

Metabolic profiles associated with normal and persistent CL progesterone profiles

PCL1 and PCL2 progesterone profiles occurred in 16% and 11% of our primiparous animals respectively. The incidence of this condition has increased from 2% (Bulman and Lamming, 1978; Bulman and Wood, 1980) to 35% in more recent investigations (1995 to 1998, Royal *et al.*, 2000) although the reason for the increase is unknown. Uterine infection is thought to interfere with the luteolytic mechanism leading to long luteal phases (Opsomer *et al.*, 1998; Wathes *et al.*, 2003). All primiparous cows that developed PCL profiles had vulval discharges and uterine involution occurred more slowly in the PCL1 cows. Compared with normal profile animals, PCL1 cows produced higher milk fat contents, had higher glucose concentrations post-calving and the lowest urea values at week 3. PCL2 cows produced higher milk fat and milk lactose contents, their IGF-I concentrations were reduced to week three of lactation and urea values were higher at week 8. All other parameters measured were similar to those of the normal profile cows. Neither group of PCL animals was in prolonged negative energy balance after calving. There may have been some metabolic differences between PCL1 and PCL2 cows, but the numbers of cows in each group were too low to draw firm conclusions. In this study on a limited number of first lactation cows the impact of a PCL profile on fertility parameters was negligible. Our multiparous HGM cow studies and the 533 cows investigated by Bulman and Wood (1980) also failed to show a significant effect of this condition on fertility parameters, although the trend was in an adverse direction. However, this ovarian condition could potentially interfere with the detection of oestrus and hence affect fertility.

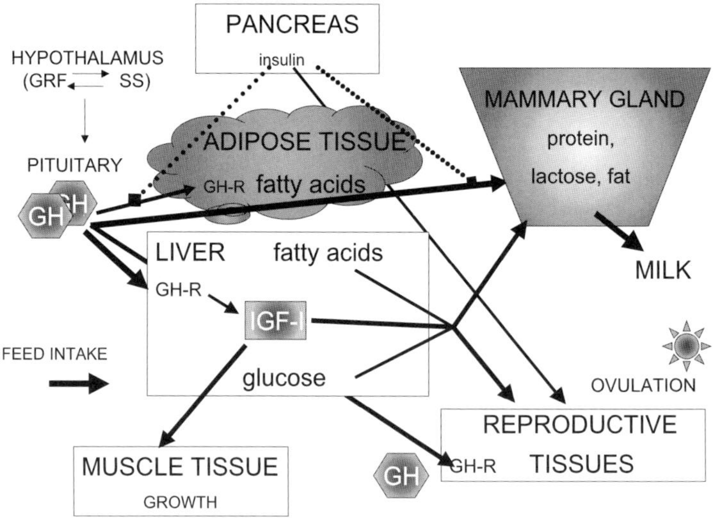

Figure 7. Proposed relationships between the somatotrophic axis, milk production and reproduction in high yielding dairy cows resulting in normal or persistent CL (PCL) progesterone profiles. See text for description.

Figure 7 summarises the proposed physiological adaptations to milk production in high yielding cows that as a consequence have either normal or persistent CL progesterone profiles. GH is secreted from the anterior pituitary, regulated by GRF and somatostatin but is also subject to negative feedback by insulin and IGF-I in an autoregulatory loop. Secreted GH promotes milk production by nutrient partitioning, increased blood flow to the mammary gland and also production of IGF-I by the liver. GH has direct effects on the ovary, stimulating growth of small follicles. IGF-I influences lean body growth and stimulates steroidogenesis in ovarian cells. Plasma glucose is sequestered for milk lactose production via insulin-insensitive glucose transporters in the mammary gland. Fatty acids in the circulation are used for both milk fat production and as a metabolic fuel in the ovary. Insulin has positive effects on lipogenesis, ovarian function and early embryo development but restrains the action of GH on adipose tissue and lipolysis. The animals with these physiological responses to lactation produce high milk yields and are also able to reproduce within the expected time frame of the management system.

Metabolic profiles associated with delayed ovulation progesterone profiles

Our primiparous DOV1 animals had higher milk energy values and milk fat contents (also found by de Vries and Veerkamp, 2000) and tended to produce less milk protein than normal profile cows (Taylor *et al.*, 2003). They also had reduced dry matter intakes (DMI) in early lactation, the lowest mean body weights and the greatest body condition score (BCS) losses post-calving than normal profile animals. These results show that the DOV1 cows were mobilising a greater amount of body tissue to support lactation and their differences in milk quality composition reflected altered nutrient partitioning. These cows reached their peak milk yields many weeks (week 9) in advance of their peak DMI (week 17) and were in prolonged negative energy balance; they also had the largest NEB values (also found by deVries, van der Beek, Kaal-Lansbergen, Ouweltjes and Wilmink, 1999). These adjustments during early lactation in DOV1 cows were also reflected in their metabolite measurements, as they had the highest BHB and numerically lowest plasma glucose concentrations in week three *post partum*, indicating a shift in metabolic fuel from glucose to fatty acids which occurs when glucose supply is limited. They also had lower concentrations of IGF-I immediately *post partum* (weeks 1 to 2) and insulin levels both before and after calving appeared to be lower, although this difference was not significant.

These metabolic data together suggest that the liver was GH resistant in DOV1 cows. High GH (as occurs *post partum*), coupled with low levels of IGF-I and insulin, could sustain milk production by promoting lipolysis in adipose tissue and ketogenesis in the liver. IGF-I, glucose and insulin values in DOV1 cows were lower immediately *post partum* but had regained similar concentrations to those in the normal profile cows by weeks 3, 5 and 6 respectively. However, the cows continued to lose condition until week 7 and did not ovulate until week 10 (median 69 days). Some previous studies have shown that excessive BCS loss was associated with a prolonged interval to first ovulation (Butler, 2000; Pryce *et al.*, 2001). Data from our larger study (Wathes *et al.*, 2001) suggest that in primiparous cows, which are still growing, insulin levels may be more limiting to reproductive function, whereas in older cows we have found a closer association between IGF-I values and fertility parameters.

Figure 8 summarises the proposed physiological adaptations to milk production in high yielding cows that as a consequence have delayed ovulation. Decreased GH-R in liver leads to GH resistance and low IGF-I concentrations immediately post-calving. This would be further exacerbated by reduced feed intake (possibly altering GH pulsatility). Low plasma glucose and fatty acids could lead to mobilisation of body reserves (muscle glycogen, muscle and adipose tissue breakdown), especially as GH actions are unrestrained by low insulin and/or IGF-I levels. GH would still act directly on the ovary promoting growth of small follicles but inadequate stimulation by insulin and IGF-I would result in ovarian dysfunction characterised by delayed ovulation. These animals may produce high milk yields but would be unable to reproduce until ovarian function is re-established.

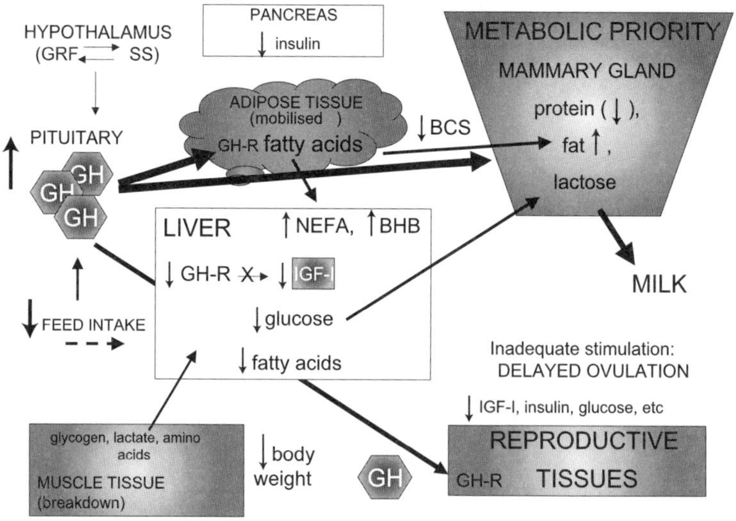

Figure 8. Proposed relationships between the somatotrophic axis, milk production and reproduction in high yielding dairy cows resulting in delayed ovulation (DOV) progesterone profiles. See text for description.

Herd and nutritional management

The reproductive performance of a dairy herd is influenced by management practises. Metabolic measurements may be more informative of an individual animal's physiological condition but single values are rarely meaningful. Using science to meet farmers' and consumers' needs requires simple and robust measures. Diagnostic reproductive measures currently being developed are online progesterone monitoring to characterise progesterone profiles (Mottram and Mason, 2001). Other investigators have suggested milk fat to protein ratios (Heuer, Schukken and Dobbelaar, 1999) and BCS at week 10 as indicators of NEB (Pryce *et al.*, 2001). Our combined data from multiparous cows (n=204) have demonstrated that very low plasma IGF-I concentrations in the early post-calving period had more influence on the possibility of a successful conception at first AI than actual IGF-I concentrations at the time of first service (Taylor, Cheng, Pushpakumara, Beever, Jones and Wathes, 2002). Our research suggests that plasma IGF-I measurement in early lactation may be a useful predictive tool for fertility in high yielding dairy cows, thus allowing cows with low concentrations of plasma IGF-I immediately post-calving and prior to first service to be identified and monitored. In a practical situation, IGF-I concentrations could be measured in two blood samples taken a) within the first week following calving and b) before the start of the service period. It is suggested that in animals with IGF-I concentrations below 25 ng/ml in week 1 post-calving and less than 50 ng/ml immediately prior to 1st service, it may be cost-effective to delay AI until IGF-I concentrations have increased to more than 50 ng/ml for a period of at least 3 weeks. Our studies have associated low IGF-I levels with failure to conceive in dairy cows. It has yet to be determined how to avoid such situations from occurring in high yielding animals but as the fall in IGF-I occurs within one week of calving, management interventions to prevent it must clearly occur well before calving.

Dietary influences on energy balance and reproductive function

Numerous studies have addressed whether different types of supplementation can improve energy or protein status of cows and hence health and productivity. Fewer studies have looked specifically at effects on reproduction and this remains an area that requires more investigation. Nutrition, especially undernutrition, arguably has the greatest impact on the whole range of fertility parameters as detailed above. Undernutrition causes uncoupling of the GH axis but overnutrition does not cause excessive IGF-I production due to the negative feedback effects of IGF-I on GH. Additionally, obesity or overconditioning causes a blunting of GH response and insulin resistance. Dietary manipulation can be targeted towards the pre-calving and the post-calving period. Many studies are undertaken in dairy cows after peak milk yields have been achieved and we suggest that it is the period prior to this that is more important in determining fertility. Thus it is not surprising that differences are not often found.

The energy and protein requirements for maintenance and pregnancy of dairy cattle increase during late gestation (Bell, 1995) but during this time feed intake usually declines. An adequate diet in the transition period is important to establish protein and energy stores in dairy cows, that are then drawn upon during early lactation (Bell, Burhans and Overton, 2000), especially body fat reserves (Beever, 2002). Bauman and Currie (1980) established that a third of the energy requirements for milk production in the first 15 weeks of lactation were derived from adipose tissue. Tamminga, Luteijn and Meijer (1997) determined that dairy cows produced an average of 324 kg milk from their body reserves during early lactation.

High protein diets in the *pre partum* period may be implicated in the development of ketosis as high levels of protein intake are associated with increased blood ketones. An 18% crude protein (CP) *pre partum* supplement appeared to stimulate ketogenesis, depress DMI and these cows lost more body condition than animals receiving a ration containing 14% CP (Putnam, Varga and Dann, 1999). There is a significant energetic cost associated with the metabolism of additional protein which may limit glucose availability. Excess crude protein and insufficient energy have been linked to suboptimal performance in terms of decreased fertility and increased days open (McCormick, French, Brown, Cuomo, Chapa, Fernandez, Beatty and Blouin, 1999), increased embryo mortality (Zavy and Geisert, 1994) and low BCS and BCS loss (Chapa, McCormick, Fernandez, French, Ward and Beatty, 2001). In contrast, low protein diets in cows were associated with reduced IGF-I by VandeHaar, Yousif, Sharma, Herdt, Emery, Allen and Liesman (1999). Methionine has been known for some time to be the first amino acid to become limiting in some forage and silage-based diets (Richardson and Hatfield, 1978) and recent work has discovered that the GH-IGF-I system in sheep is selectively sensitive to its presence (Stubbs *et al.*, 2002). The addition of bST may increase IGF-I concentrations; however its use is likely to limit an animal's ability to re-gain body-weight and BCS, especially in lactation. Fat supplements have been given to early lactation dairy cows to increase EB but with inconsistent results (Spicer *et al.*, 1993; Beam and Butler, 1999). Some improvements in reproductive function (return to cyclicity, conception rates and days open) have been found in prepartum fat supplemented multiparous cows (Reynolds, Jones, Phipps, Dürst, Lupoli and Aikman, 2002). Dietary means of increasing *post partum* insulin concentrations include promoting ruminal propionate production (Landau, Bor, Leibovich, Zoref and Nitsan, 1995), eg using glycogenic agents such as propylene glycol (Grummer, Winkler, Bertics and Studer, 1994; Miyoshi, Pate and Palmquist, 2001), increasing dietary protein (Landau, Braw-Tal, Kaim, Bor and Bruckental, 2000) but in some cases, when fed over long time-periods this may have a detrimental effect on feed intake. Increased insulin concentrations are also antagonistic to milk production (Hart *et al.*, 1978). Whilst varying responses have been observed in studies investigating dietary modifications, Beever (2002) has identified four key priorities for dairy herd management: (1) an uneventful calving with no associated metabolic disorders; (2) rapid establishment of satisfactory levels of feed intake; (3) minimisation of body energy mobilisation and (4) establishment of reproductive cyclicity followed by a successful pregnancy.

Short term nutritional improvements, raising plasma and intrafollicular concentrations of IGF-I and other growth factors and optimising insulin and glucose levels, targeted towards specific reproductive events may be of practical importance in improving fertility in high yielding dairy cows. However, making nutritional changes at AI is not advisable as the rumen micro flora need time to adjust to dietary changes. There are also likely to be different requirements for primiparous and multiparous cows. Short term aims should be to avoid GH resistance occurring from situations such as undernutrition caused by reduced DMI and diseases such as mastitis and endometritis. Longer term aims should be to devise nutritional and/or management strategies to avoid the occurrence of GH resistance. Only when we have a better understanding of the causes of physiological adaptations to milk yield and their effects on fertility can such information be incorporated into genetic selection programmes.

Conclusions

Our studies revealed that, whilst associated with high milk yields, not all progesterone profile categories detrimentally affected fertility parameters and the incidences were different between primiparous and multiparous cows. The occurrence of ovarian dysfunction may be an appropriate response to a nutritional state or physiological situation. Delayed ovulation appears to occur when body reserves are mobilised to maintain milk yields at the expense of reproduction and seems most likely to occur in primiparous high yielding cows or those experiencing GH-resistance (low IGF-I) due to excessive body condition loss, reduced feed intakes and factors such as stress and disease. Despite the increasing incidence of persistent luteal phases (PCLs) in dairy cows, this condition was not found to have any substantial detrimental effects on fertility or production parameters of the primiparous or multiparous cows in these studies. The major reproductive problems in our high yielding primiparous and multiparous cows appeared to be a failure to ovulate and conceive at the expected time or to maintain a pregnancy. These situations were associated predominantly with high milk yields and low concentrations of plasma IGF-I and insulin. More detailed investigations of dietary means of increasing IGF-I and optimising insulin concentrations, targeted at important reproductive times are required in high yielding dairy cows, to aid in their management.

Acknowledgements

The authors are grateful to the staff at the Animal Production Research Unit and the Centre for Dairy Research, University of Reading for the care of the animals. Thanks are due to Mrs Ailiang Zhang for analysis of some samples. This work was funded by the Milk Development Council (MDC) and DEFRA.

References

Armstrong, J.D., Cohick, W.S., Harvey, R.W., Heimer, E.P. and Campbell, R.M. (1993) Effect of feed restriction on serum somatotropin, insulin-like growth factor-I (IGF-I) and IGF binding proteins in cyclic heifers actively immunized against growth hormone releasing factor. *Domestic Animal Endocrinology* **10**, 315-324.

Armstrong, J.D., Coffey, M.T., Esbenshade, K.L., Campbell, R.M. and Heimer, E.P. (1994) Concentrations of hormones and metabolites, estimates of metabolism, performance, and reproductive performance of sows actively immunized against growth hormone-releasing factor. *Journal of Animal Science* **72**, 1570-1577.

Bagnato, A. and Oltenacu, P.A. (1994) Phenotypic evaluation of fertility traits and their association with milk production of Italian Friesian cattle. *Journal of Dairy Science* **77**, 874-882.

Bartke, A., Chandrashekar, V., Turyn, D., Steger, R.W., Debeljuk, L., Winters, T.A., Mattison, J.A., Danilovich, N.A., Croson, W., Wernsing, D.R. and Kopchick, J.J. (1999) Effects of growth hormone overexpression and growth hormone resistance on neuroendocrine and reproductive functions in transgenic and knock-out mice. *Proceedings of the Society for Experimental Biology and Medicine* **222**, 113-123.

Bauman, D.E. and Currie, W.B. (1980) Partitioning of nutrients during pregnancy and lactation: a review of mechanisms involving homeostasis and homeorhesis. *Journal of Dairy Science* **63**, 1514-1529.

Beam, S.W. and Butler, W.R. (1999) Effects of energy balance on follicular development and first ovulation in postpartum dairy cows. *Journal of Reproduction and Fertility Supplement* **54**, 411-424.

Beever, D.E., Hattan, A., Reynolds, C.K. and Cammell, S.B. (2001) Nutrient supply to high-yielding dairy cows. Fertility in the High-Producing Dairy Cow, British Society of Animal Science Occasional Publication No. 26, Volume 1, 119-131.

Beever, D.E. (2002) *Nutritional Management of the Transition Cow.* CEDAR Report No. 179 for the Milk Development Council.

Bell, A.W. (1995) Regulation of organic nutrient metabolism during transition from late pregnancy to early lactation. *Journal of Animal Science* **73**, 2804-2819.

Bell, A.W., Burhans, W.S. and Overton, T.R. (2000) Protein nutrition in late pregnancy, maternal protein reserves and lactation performance in dairy cows. *Proceedings of the Nutrition Society* **59**, 119-126.

Berry, D.P., Buckley, F., Dillon, P., Evans, R.D., Rath, M. and Veerkamp R.F. (2002) Genetic parameters for level and change of body condition score and body weight in dairy cows. *Journal of Dairy Science* **85**, 2030-2039.

Bonczek, R.R., Young, C.W., Wheaton, J.E. and Miller, K.P. (1988) Response of somatotropin, insulin, prolactin and thyroxine to selection for milk yield in Holsteins. *Journal of Dairy Science* **71**, 2470-2479.

Brown-Borg, H.M., Rakoczy, S.G., Romanick, M.A. and Kennedy, M. (2002) A.Effects of growth hormone and insulin-like growth factor-1 on hepatocyte antioxidative enzymes. *Experimental Biology and Medicine* **227**, 94-104.

Bulman, D.C. and Lamming, G.E. (1978) Milk progesterone levels in relation to conception, repeat breeding and factors influencing acyclicity in dairy cows. *Journal of Reproduction and Fertility* **54**, 447-458.

Bulman, D.C. and Wood, P.D.P. (1980) Abnormal patterns of ovarian activity in dairy cows and their relationships with reproductive performance. *Animal Production* **30**, 177-188.

Butler, W.R. (2000) Nutritional interactions with reproductive performance in dairy cattle. *Animal Reproduction Science* **60-61**, 449-457.

Butler, W.R. and Smith, R.D. (1989) Interrelationships between energy balance and postpartum reproductive function in dairy cattle. *Journal of Dairy Science* **72**, 767-783.

Chapa, A.M., McCormick, M.E., Fernandez, J.M., French, D.D., Ward, J.D. and Beatty, J.F. (2001) Supplemental dietary protein for grazing dairy cows: reproduction, condition loss, plasma metabolites, and insulin. *Journal of Dairy Science* **84**, 908-916.

Chase Jr, C.C., Kirby, C.J., Hammond, A.C., Olson, T.A.and Lucy, M.C. (1998) Patterns of ovarian growth and development in cattle with a growth hormone receptor deficiency. *Journal of Animal Science* **76**, 212-219.

Childs, G.V. (2000) Growth hormone cells as co-gonadotropes: partners in the regulation of the reproductive system. *Trends in Endocrinology and Metabolism* **11**, 168-175.

Clark, R. (1997) The somatogenic hormones and insulin-like growth factor-1: stimulators of lymphopoiesis and immune function. *Endocrine Reviews* **18**, 157-179.

Danilovich, N.A., Bartke, A. and Winters, T.A. (2000) Ovarian follicle apoptosis in bovine growth hormone transgenic mice. *Biology of Reproduction* **62**, 103-107.

Darwash, A.O. and Lamming, G.E. (1997) Abnormal ovarian patterns as a cause of subfertility in dairy cows: protocols for early detection and treatment. *Cattle Practice* **5**, 3-7.

Davoren, J.B. and Hsueh, A.J. (1986) Growth hormone increases ovarian levels of immunoreactive somatomedin C/insulin-like growth factor

I in vivo. *Endocrinology* **118**, 888-890.
de Vries, M.J. and Veerkamp, R.F. (2000) Energy balance of dairy cattle in relation to milk production variables and fertility. *Journal of Dairy Science* **83**, 62-69.
de Vries, M.J., van der Beek, S., Kaal-Lansbergen, L.M., Ouweltjes, W. and Wilmink, J.B. (1999) Modeling of energy balance in early lactation and the effect of energy deficits in early lactation on first detected estrus postpartum in dairy cows. *Journal of Dairy Science* **82**, 1927-1934.
Dominici, F.P. and Turyn, D. (2002) Growth hormone-induced alterations in the insulin-signaling system. *Exp Biol Med.* **227**, 149-157.
Einspanier, R., Miyamoto, A., Schams, D., Muller, M. and Brem, G. (1990) Tissue concentration, mRNA expression and stimulation of IGF-I in luteal tissue during the oestrous cycle and pregnancy of cows. *Journal of Reproduction and Fertility* **90**, 439-445.
Eisenhauer, K.M., Chun, S.Y., Billig, H. and Hsueh, A.J. (1995) Growth hormone suppression of apoptosis in preovulatory rat follicles and partial neutralization by insulin-like growth factor binding protein. *Biology of Reproduction* **53**, 13-20.
Esteban, E., Kass, P.H., Weaver, L.D., Rowe, J.D., Holmberg, C.A., Franti, C.E. and Troutt, H.F. (1994) Pregnancy incidence in high producing dairy cows treated with recombinant bovine somatotropin. *Journal of Dairy Science* **77**, 468-481.
Etherton, T.D. and Bauman, D.E. (1998) Biology of somatotropin in growth and lactation of domestic animals. *Physiological Reviews* **78**, 745-761.
Fliesen, T., Maiter, D., Gerard, G., Underwood, L.E., Maes, M. and Ketelslegers, J.M. (1989) Reduction of serum insulin-like growth factor-I by dietary protein restriction is age dependent. *Pediatric Research* **26**, 415-419.
Gatford, K.L., Egan, A.R., Clarke, I.J. and Owens, P.C. (1998) Sexual dimorphism of the somatotropic axis. *Journal of Endocrinology* **157**, 373-389.
Gracia-Navarro, F., Castano, J.P., Malagon, M.M., Sanchez-Hormigo, A., Luque, R.M., Hickey, G.J., Peinado, J.R., Delgado, E. and Martinez-Fuentes, A.J. (2002) Research progress in the stimulatory inputs regulating growth hormone (GH) secretion. *Comparative Biochemistry and Physiology. Part B, Biochemistry and Molecular Biology* **132**, 141-150.
Grochowska, R., Sorensen, P., Zwierzchowski, L., Snochowski, M. and Lovendahl, P. (2001) Genetic variation in stimulated GH release and in IGF-I of young dairy cattle and their associations with the leucine/valine polymorphism in the GH gene. *Journal of Animal Science* **79**, 470-476.
Grummer, R.R., Winkler, J.C., Bertics, S.J. and Studer, V.A. (1994) Effect of propylene glycol dosage during feed restriction on metabolites in blood of prepartum Holstein heifers. *Journal of*

Dairy Science 77, 3618-3623.

Hammond, J.M., Mondschein, J.S., Samaras, S.E., Smith, S.A. and Hagen, D.R. (1991) The ovarian insulin-like growth factor system. *Journal of Reproduction and Fertility Supplement* 43, 199-208.

Hansen, L.B., Freeman, A.E. and Berger, P.J. (1983) Association of heifer fertility with cow fertility and yield in dairy cattle. *Journal of Dairy Science* 66, 306-314.

Harrison, R.O., Ford, S.P., Young, J.W., Conley, A.J. and Freeman, A.E. (1990) Increased milk production versus reproductive and energy status of high producing dairy cows. *Journal of Dairy Science* 73, 2749-2758.

Hart, I.C., Flux, D.S., Andrews, P. and McNeilly, A.S. (1978) Endocrine control of energy metabolism in the cow: comparison of the levels of hormones (prolactin, growth hormone, insulin and thyroxine) and metabolites in the plasma of high- and low-yielding cattle at various stages of lactation. *Journal of Endocrinolgy* 77, 333-345.

Hayashida, T., Murakami, K., Mogi, K., Nishihara, M., Nakazato, M., Mondal, M.S., Horii, Y., Kojima, M., Kangawa, K. and Murakami, N. (2001) Ghrelin in domestic animals: distribution in stomach and its possible role. *Domestic Animal Endocrinology* 21, 17-24.

Heuer, C., Schukken, Y.H. and Dobbelaar, P. (1999) Postpartum body condition score and results from the first test day milk as predictors of disease, fertility, yield, and culling in commercial dairy herds. *Journal of Dairy Science* 82, 295-304.

Hoekstra, J., van der Lugt, A.W., van der Werf, J.H.J. and Ouweltjes, W. (1994) Genetic and phenotypic parameters for milk production and fertility traits in upgraded dairy cattle. *Livestock Reproduction Science* 40, 225-232.

Hossner, K.L., McCusker, R.H. and Dodson, M.V. (1997) Insulin-like growth factors and their binding proteins in domestic animals. *Animal Science* 64, 1-15.

Hugues, J.N., Miro, F., Smyth, C.D. and Hillier, S.G. (1996) Effects of growth hormone-releasing hormone on rat ovarian steroidogenesis. *Human Reproduction* 11, 50-54.

Kendrick, K.W., Bailey, T.L., Garst, A.S., Pryor, A.W., Ahmadzadeh, A., Akers, R.M., Eyestone, W.E., Pearson, R.E. and Gwazdauskas, F.C. (1999) Effects of energy balance of hormones, ovarian activity, and recovered oocytes in lactating Holstein cows using transvaginal follicular aspiration. *Journal of Dairy Science* 82, 1731-1741.

Kinsel, M.L., Marsh, W.E., Ruegg, P.L. and Etherington, W.G. (1998) Risk factors for twinning in dairy cows. *Journal of Dairy Science* 81, 989-993.

Kirby, C.J., Thatcher, W.W., Collier, R.J., Simmen, F.A. and Lucy, M.C. (1996) Effects of growth hormone and pregnancy on expression of growth hormone receptor, insulin-like growth factor-I and insulin-like growth factor binding protein-2 and -3 genes in bovine uterus, ovary and oviduct. *Biology of Reproduction* 55, 996-1002.

Kojima, M., Hosoda, H., Matsuo, H. and Kangawa, K. (2001) Ghrelin: discovery of the natural endogenous ligand for the growth hormone secretagogue receptor. *Trends in Endocrinology and Metabolism* 12, 118-122.

Kölle, S., Sinowatz, F., Boie, G., Lincoln, D. and Waters, M.J. (1997) Differential expression of the growth hormone receptor and its transcript in bovine uterus and placenta. *Molecular and Cellular Endocrinology* 131, 127-136.

Kölle, S., Sinowatz, F., Boie, G. and Lincoln, D. (1998a) Developmental changes in the expression of the growth hormone receptor messenger ribonucleic acid and protein in the bovine ovary. *Biology of Reproduction* 59, 836-842.

Kölle, S., Sinowatz, F., Boie, G., Lincoln, D., Palma, G., Stojkovic, M. and Wolf, E. (1998b) Topography of growth hormone receptor expression in the bovine embryo. *Histochemistry and Cell Biology* 109, 417-419.

Lamming, G.E. and Darwash, A.O. (1998) The use of milk progesterone profiles to characterise components of subfertility in milked dairy cows. *Animal Reproduction Science* 52, 175-190.

Lamming, G.E., Darwash, A.O., Wathes, D.C. and Ball, P.J. (1998) The fertility of dairy cattle in the UK: current status and future research. *Journal of the Royal Agricultural Society* 159, 82-93.

Lamming, G.E. and Royal, M.D. (2001) Ovarian hormone patterns and sub fertility in dairy cows. *Fertility in the High-Producing Dairy Cow*, British Society of Animal Science Occasional Publication No. 26, 1, 105-118.

Landau, S.Bor, A., Leibovich, H., Zoref, Z. and Nitsan, Z. (1995) The effect of ruminal starch degradability in the diet of crossbred ewes on induced ovulation rate and prolificacy. *Animal Reproduction Science* 38, 97-108.

Landau, S., Braw-Tal, R., Kaim, M., Bor, A. and Bruckental, I.I. (2000) Preovulatory follicular status and diet affect the insulin and glucose content of follicles in high-yielding dairy cows. *Animal Reproduction Science* 64,181-197.

Lang, C.H. and Frost, R.A. (2002) Role of growth hormone, insulin-like growth factor-I, and insulin-like growth factor binding proteins in the catabolic response to injury and infection. *Current Opinions in Clinical Nutrition and Metabolic Care* 5, 271-279.

Leeuwenberg, B.R., Hudson, N.L., Moore, L.G., Hurst, P.R. and McNatty, K.P. (1996) Peripheral and ovarian IGF-I concentrations during the ovine oestrous cycle. *Journal of Endocrinology* 148, 281-289.

Lindhé, B. and Philipsson, J. (2001) The Scandinavian experience of including reproductive traits in breeding programmes. *Fertility in the High-Producing Dairy Cow*, British Society of Animal Science Occasional Publication No. 26, Volume 1, 251-261.

Lucy, M.C., Staples, C.R., Michel, F.M. and Thatcher, W.W. (1991) Energy balance and size and number of ovarian follicles detected by ultrasonography in early postpartum dairy cows. *Journal of Dairy Science* 74, 473-482.

Lucy, M.C., Hauser, S.D., Eppard, P.J., Krivi, G.G., Clark, J.H., Bauman, D.E. and Collier, R.J. (1993) Variants of somatotropin in cattle: gene frequencies in major dairy breeds and associated milk production. *Domestic Animal Endocrinology* **10**, 325-333.

Lucy, M.C., Boyd, C.K., Koenigsfeld, A.T. and Okamura, C.S. (1998) Expression of somatotropin receptor messenger ribonucleic acid in bovine tissues. *Journal of Dairy Science* **81**, 1889-1895.

Mackey, D.R., Sreenan, J.M., Roche, J.F. and Diskin, M.G. (1999) Effect of acute nutritional restriction on incidence of anovulation and periovulatory estradiol and gonadotropin concentrations in beef heifers. *Biology of Reproduction* **61**, 1601-1607.

McCormick M.E., French, D.D., Brown, T.F., Cuomo, G.J., Chapa, A.M., Fernandez, J.M., Beatty, J.F. and Blouin, D.C. (1999) Crude protein and rumen undergradable protein effects on reproduction and lactation performance of Holstein cows. *Journal of Dairy Science* **82**, 2697-2708.

McCusker, R.H. (1998) Controlling insulin-like growth factor activity and the modulation of insulin-like growth factor binding protein and receptor binding. *Journal of Dairy Science* **81**, 1790-1800.

McGuire, M.A., Vicini, J.L., Bauman, D.E. and Veenhuizen, J.J. (1992) Insulin-like growth factors and binding proteins in ruminants and their nutritional regulation. *Journal of Animal Science* **70**, 2901-2910.

McGuire, M.A., Dywer, D.A., Harrell, R.J. and Bauman, D.E. (1995) Insulin regulates circulating insulin-like growth factors and some of their binding proteins in lactating cows. *American Journal of Physiology* **269**, E723-730.

Minegishi, T., Hirakawa, T., Kishi, H., Abe, K., Abe, Y., Mizutani, T. and Miyamoto, K. (2000) A role of insulin-like growth factor I for follicle-stimulating hormone receptor expression in rat granulosa cells. *Biology of Reproduction* **62**, 325-333.

Miyoshi, S., Pate, J.L. and Palmquist, D.L. (2001) Effects of propylene glycol drenching on energy balance, plasma glucose, plasma insulin, ovarian function and conception in dairy cows. *Animal Reproduction Science* **68**, 29-43.

Mottram, T.T. and Masson, L. (2001) Dumb animals and smart machines: the implications of modern milking systems for integrated management of dairy cows. Integrated Management Systems for Livestock Production, British Society of Animal Science Occasional Publication No. **28**, 77-84.

Murphy, M.G., Enright, W.J., Crowe, M.A., McConnell, K., Spicer,

L.J., Boland, M.P. and Roche, J.F. (1991) Effect of dietary intake on pattern of growth of dominant follicles during the oestrous cycle in beef heifers. *Journal of Reproduction and Fertility* 92, 333-338.

Nam, S.Y. and Lobie, P.E. (2000) The mechanism of effect of growth hormone on preadipocyte and adipocyte function. *Obesity Reviews* 1, 73-86.

Nebel, R.L. and McGilliard, M.L. (1993) Interactions of high milk yield and reproductive performance in dairy cows. *Journal of Dairy Science* 76, 3257-3268.

Nielsen, B.L., Veerkamp, R.F., Pryce, J.E., Simm, G. and Oldham, J.D. (1997) Effects of genotype and lactation number on health and reproductive problems in dairy cows. Proceedings of the British Society of Animal Science (Abstracts), 143.

Opsomer, G., Coryn, M., Deluyker, H. and de Kruif, A. (1998) An analysis of ovarian dysfunction in high yielding dairy cows after calving based on progesterone profiles. *Reproduction in Domestic Animals* 33, 193-204.

Osgerby, J.C., Gadd, T.S. and Wathes, D.C. (1999) Expression of insulin-like growth factor binding protein-1 (IGFBP-1) mRNA in the ovine uterus throughout the oestrous cycle and early pregnancy. *Journal of Endocrinology* 162, 279-287.

Parks, J.S. (2001) The ontogeny of growth hormone sensitivity. *Hormone Research* 55, Supplement 2, 27-31.

Perks, C.M., Peters, A.R. and Wathes, D.C. (1999) Follicular and luteal expression of insulin-like growth factors I and II and the type 1 IGF receptor in the bovine ovary. *Journal of Reproduction and Fertility* 116, 157-165.

Pryce, J.E., Veerkamp, R.F., Thompson, R., Hill, W.G. and Simm, G. (1997) Genetic aspects of common health disorders and measures of fertility in Holstein Friesian dairy cattle. *Animal Science* 65, 353-360.

Pryce, J.E., Esslemont, R.J., Thompson, R., Veerkamp, R.F., Kossaibati, M.A. and Simm, G. (1998) Estimation of genetic parameters using health, fertility and production data from a management recording system for dairy cattle. *Animal Science* 66, 577-584.

Pryce, J.E., Nielsen, B.L., Veerkamp, R.F. and Simm, G. (1999) Genotype and feeding system effects and interactions for health and fertility traits in dairy cattle. *Livestock Production Science* 57, 193-201.

Pryce, J.E., Coffey, M.P. and Brotherstone, S. (2000) The genetic relationship between calving interval, body condition score and linear type and management traits in registered Holsteins. *Journal of Dairy Science* 83, 2664-2671.

Pryce, J.E., Coffey, M.P. and Simm, G. (2001) The relationship between body condition score and reproductive performance. *Journal of Dairy Science* 84, 1508-1515.

Pushpakumara, P.G.A., Robinson, R.S., Demmers, K.J., Mann, G.E., Sinclair, K.D., Webb, R. and Wathes, D.C. (2002) Expression of the insulin-like growth factor (IGF) system in the bovine oviduct at oestrus and during early pregnancy. *Reproduction* 123, 859-868.

Putnam, D.E., Varga, G.A. and Dann, H.M. (1999) Metabolic and production responses to dietary protein and exogenous somatotropin in late gestation dairy cows. *Journal of Dairy Science* 82, 982-995.

Reynolds, C.K., Jones, A.K., Phipps, R.H., Dürst, B., Lupoli, B. and Aikman, P.C. (2002) Nutritional Management of the Transition Cow for Optimal Health and Production. Part 1. Production, reproductive and metabolic responses to supplemental concentrates during the dry period – lactation trials. CEDAR Report No. 176, Milk Development Council.

Richardson, C.R. and Hatfield, E.E. (1978) The limiting amino acids in growing cattle. *Journal of Animal Science* **46**, 740-745.

Robinson, R.S., Mann, G.E., Gadd, T.S., Lamming, G.E. and Wathes, D.C. (2000) The expression of the IGF system in the bovine uterus throughout the oestrous cycle and early pregnancy. *Journal of Endocrinology* **165**, 231-243.

Ronge, H., Blum, J., Clement, C., Jans, F., Leuenberger, H. and Binder, H. (1988) Somatomedin C in dairy cows related to energy and protein supply and to milk production. *Animal Production* **47**, 165-183.

Royal, M.D., Darwash, A.O., Flint, A.P.F., Webb, R., Woolliams, J.A. and Lamming, G.E. (2000) Declining fertility in dairy cattle: changes in traditional and endocrine parameters of fertility. *Animal Science* **70**, 487-501.

Sauerwein, H., Miyamoto, A., Gunther, J., Meyer, H.H. and Schams, D. (1992) Binding and action of insulin-like growth factors and insulin in bovine luteal tissue during the oestrous cycle. *Journal of Reproduction and Fertility* **96**, 103-115.

Savage, M.O., Burren, C.P. Blair, J.C., Woods, K.A., Metherell, L., Clark, A.J. and Camacho-Hubner, C. (2001) Growth hormone insensitivity: pathophysiology, diagnosis, clinical variation and future perspectives. *Hormone Research* **55**, Supplement 2, 32-35.

Schlee, P., Graml, R., Schallenberger, E., Schams, D., Rottman, O., Olbrich-Bludau, A. and Pirchner, F. (1994) Growth hormone and insulin-like growth factor I concentrations in bulls of various growth hormone genotypes. *Theoretical and Applied Genetics* **88**, 497-500.

Schoppee, P.D., Armstrong, J.D., Harvey, R.W., Whitacre, M.D., Felix, A. and Campbell, R.M. (1996) Immunization against growth hormone-releasing factor or chronic feed restriction initiated at 3.5 months of age reduces ovarian response to pulsatile administration of gonadotropin-releasing hormone at 6 months of age and delays onset of puberty in heifers. *Biology of Reproduction* 55, 87-98.

Senatore, E.M., Butler, W.R. and Oltenacu, P.A. (1996) Relationships between energy balance and post-partum ovarian activity and fertility in first lactation dairy cows. *Animal Science* 62, 17-23.

Sirotkin, A.V., Chrenek, P., Makarevich, A.V., Huba, J. and Bulla, J. (2000) Interrelationships between breed, growth hormone genotype, plasma IGF-I level and meat performance in bulls of different ages. *Archiv für Tierzucht* 43, 591-596.

Snijders, S.E.M., Dillon, P.G., O'Callaghan, D. and Boland, M.P. (2000) Effect of genetic merit, milk yield, body condition and lactation number on in vitro oocyte development in dairy cows. *Theriogenology* 53, 981-989.

Sørensen, P., Grochowska, R., Holm, L., Henryon, M. and Løvendahl P. (2002) Polymorphism in the Bovine Growth Hormone Gene Affects Endocrine Release in Dairy Calves. *Journal of Dairy Science* 85,1887-1893.

Spicer, L.J., Alpizar, E. and Echternkamp, S.E. (1993) Effects of insulin, insulin-like growth factor I, and gonadotropins on bovine granulosa cell proliferation, progesterone production, estradiol production, and(or) insulin-like growth factor I production in vitro. *Journal of Animal Science* 71, 1232-1241.

Spicer, L.J. and Echternkamp, S.E. (1995) The ovarian insulin and insulin-like growth factor system with an emphasis on domestic animals. *Domestic Animal Endocrinology* 12, 223-245.

Sreenan, J.M. and Diskin, M.G. (1983) Early embryonic mortality in the cow: its relationship with progesterone concentration. *Veterinary Record* 112, 517-521.

Staples, C.R., Burke, J.M. and Thatcher, W.W. (1998) Influence of supplemental fats on reproductive tissues and performance of lactating cows. *Journal of Dairy Science* 81, 856-871.

Stubbs, A.K., Wheelhouse, N.M., Lomax, M.A. and Hazlerigg, D.G. (2002) Nutrient-hormone interaction in the ovine liver: methionine supply selectively modulates growth hormone-induced IGF-I gene expression. *Journal of Endocrinology* 174, 335-341.

Tamminga, S., Luteijn and Meijer, R.G.M. (1997) Changes in composition and energy content of liveweight loss in dairy cows with time after parturition. *Livestock Reproduction Science* 52, 31-38.

Taylor, V.J., Beever, D.E., Bryant, M.J. and Wathes, D.C. (2003) Metabolic profiles and progesterone cycles in first lactation dairy cows. *Theriogenology* 59, 1661-1677.

Taylor, V.J., Cheng, Z., Pushpakumara, P.G.A., Beever, D.E., Jones, A.K. and Wathes, D.C. (2002) Fertility in lactating dairy cows:diagnostic value of plasma IGF-I. *6th International Symposium on Reproduction in Domestic Ruminants*. A79.

Taylor, V.J., Hattan, A.J., Bleach, E.C.L., Beever, D.E. and Wathes, D.C. (2001) Reproductive function in average and high yielding dairy cows. Fertility in the High-Producing Dairy Cow, British Society of Animal Science Occasional Publication No. 26, Volume 2, 495-498.

Thatcher, W.W. and Wilcox, C.J. (1973) Postpartum estrus as an indicator of reproductive status in the dairy cow. *Journal of Dairy Science* 56, 608-610.

Thissen, J-P., Ketelslegers, J-M. and Underwood, L.E. (1994) Nutritional regulation of the insulin-like growth factors. *Endocrine Reviews* 15, 80-101.

VandeHaar, M.J., Yousif, G., Sharma, B.K., Herdt, T.H., Emery, R.S., Allen, M.S. and Liesman, J.S. (1999) Effect of energy and protein density of prepartum diets on fat and protein metabolism of dairy cattle in the periparturient period. *Journal of Dairy Science* 82, 1282-1295.

Veldhuis, J.D., Anderson, S.M., Shah, N., Bray, M., Vick, T., Gentili, A., Mulligan, T., Johnson, M.L., Weltman, A., Evans, W.S. and Iranmanesh, A. (2001) Neurophysiological regulation and target-tissue impact of the pulsatile mode of growth hormone secretion in the human. *Growth Hormone and IGF Research* 11, Supplement A, S25-37.

Vesela, J., Cikos, S., Hlinka, D., Rehak, P., Baran, V.and Koppel, J. (1995) Effects of impaired insulin secretion on the fertilization of mouse oocytes. *Human Reproduction* 10, 3233-3236.

Wandji, S.A., Gadsby, J.E., Simmen, F.A., Barber, J.A. and Hammond, J.M. (2000) Porcine ovarian cells express messenger ribonucleic acids for the acid-labile subunit and insulin-like growth factor binding protein-3 during follicular and luteal phases of the estrous cycle. *Endocrinology* 141, 2638-2647.

Wathes, D.C., Perks, C.M., Davis, A.J. and Denning-Kendall, P.A. (1995) Regulation of insulin-like growth factor-I and progesterone synthesis by insulin and growth hormone in the ovine ovary. *Biology of Reproduction* 53, 882-889.

Wathes, D.C., Beever, D.E., Cheng, Z., Pushpakumara, P.G.A. and Taylor, V.J. (2001) Life-time organisation and management of reproduction in the dairy cow. Integrated Management Systems for Livestock Production, British Society of Animal Science Occasional Publication No. 28, 59-69.

Wathes, D.C., Taylor, V.J., Cheng, Z. and Mann, G.E. (2003) Follicle growth, corpus luteum function and their effects on embryo development in postpartum dairy cows. Reproduction in Domestic Ruminants V. Reproduction Supplement 61: 219-237, Cambridge University Press.

Zavy, M.T. and Geisert, R.D. (1994) Embryonic Mortality in Domestic Species. CRC Press, Boca Raton, Florida, USA.

3

METABOLIC CONSEQUENCES OF INCREASING MILK YIELD – REVISITING LORNA

C. K. Reynolds
Department of Animal Sciences, The Ohio State University, OARDC, Wooster, Ohio, 44691, USA.

Introduction

Nearly 50 years ago, a cow named Lorna achieved notoriety by producing nearly 50 kg of milk daily during measurements of her energy metabolism in a calorimeter at the United States Department of Agriculture (USDA) Energy Metabolism Laboratory at Beltsville, Maryland (Flatt, Moore, Hooven and Plowman, 1965; Flatt, Moe, Munson and Cooper, 1969). In the intervening period genetic selection in dairy cattle has produced huge increases in average milk yield, as well as changes in overall conformation, udder characteristics, and body size and structure (Hansen, 2000). Increases in annual milk yield by the total US dairy herd continue at much the same pace as has occurred for the last 50 years (Figure 1; www.usda.gov/nass), with no sign that limits of production capacity or biological efficiency have been reached (Figure 2; www.aipl.arsusda.gov). In actual fact, the increase in breeding value for milk yield has been accelerating during the same time period (Hansen, 2000). The current record for milk yield, as far as I am aware, stands at nearly 31,000 kg for 365 days, by a cow milked twice daily (www.holsteinusa.com). Does this represent a metabolic or physical ceiling? Based on genetic trends (Figure 2), it is highly likely this record will some day be broken, whilst the average yield of 'normal' cows catches up with the old record holder in the intervening period. How have these increases in milk yield been achieved? Are 'modern' high yielding dairy cows metabolically different from Lorna and her contemporaries in 1964?

In many countries, changes in cow genetics have accompanied the evolution of dairy farming from a 'livelihood' to a 'business' and now fewer cows produce more milk (Figure 1) on fewer farms. In the USA, the number of milk cow operations has decreased by a staggering 43% in the last 10 years, to under 100,000 (www.usda.gov/nass). This evolution has been driven by a variety of economic, social and political pressures, but is often justified on the basis of economy of scale and dilution of fixed costs. Whilst many dairy farmers see milk yield as a yardstick of their ability as herd managers, economic success is the bottom line of job performance, and profit, or survival, is a balance between outputs and inputs. In the USA, harvesting and handling costs often mean that conserved forage is a more expensive component of dairy rations than concentrates, as corn and other co-product feeds are abundant. In countries where grain is more expensive, and even in sectors of the US dairy industry, economic, social and political pressure has led to the evolution of so called 'low input' dairy management systems, such as those based on grazed grass. Thus in the UK, and other countries where grass is the backbone of the dairy industry, the suitability of North American (NA) genetics, and the implications of increasing milk yield, have been the subject of considerable discussion, and a number of recent symposia (e.g. www.bsas.org/publs). Concerns include the effects of high milk yield on levels of 'metabolic stress', the welfare of the cow, her ability to reproduce, her 'longevity', and ultimately her lifetime production. Other papers will consider reproduction and longevity in more detail. This paper will consider metabolic implications of increased milk yield for the dairy cow, and potential interactions with management environment, but not the economic implications for the dairy enterprise. Using Lorna and her contemporaries as a point of reference, I will consider how the high yielding dairy cow has, or has not, changed over the last 50 years.

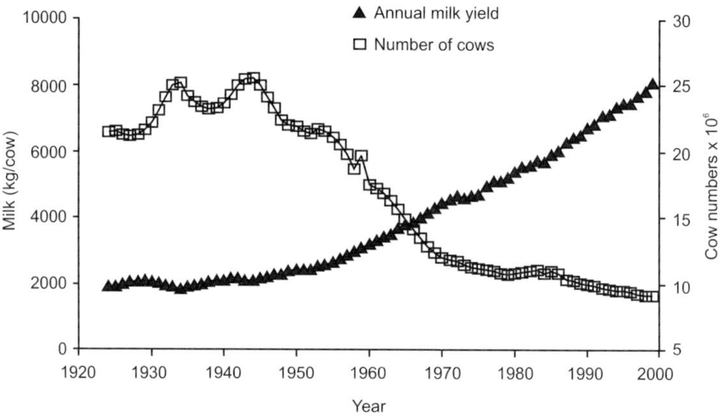

Figure 1. Annual milk yield and cow numbers in the USA from 1924 to 1999 (www.usda.gov/nass).

Achieving greater milk yield

How has selection for greater milk yield changed the dairy cow metabolically? Energetically, increases in milk yield can only be achieved in one of 3 ways. Firstly, does she simply consume, or acquire, more metabolisable energy (ME) from her feed? Secondly, is she more efficient in using ME from her feed for milk energy? Finally, does she loose more body energy stores (condition) to support milk yield?

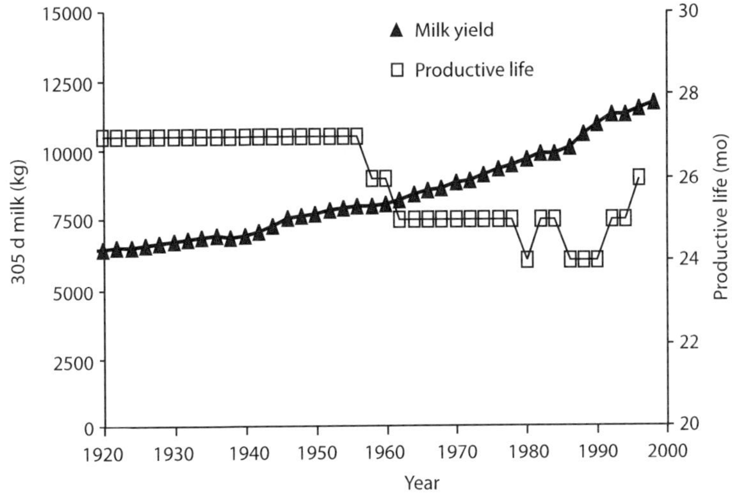

Figure 2. Breeding value for milk yield and productive life in US Holsteins (www.aipl.arsusda.gov).

Feed intake

Copious milk production requires a copious supply of nutrients for milk synthesis, and thus nutrient requirements, appetite, and feed intake capacity have increased in tandem with milk yield. In a number of comparisons of production data from low- and high-yielding genetic lines of dairy cows (Gordon, Patterson, Yan, Porter, Mayne and Unsworth, 1995; Veerkamp, Simm and Oldham, 1995; Crooker, Weber, Ma and Lucy, 1999; Buckley, Dillon, Rath and Veerkamp, 2000), higher yielding lines consume more feed, which is in part a consequence of greater appetite and selection for physical and perhaps physiological characteristics which may allow more feed intake. There is no evidence to suggest that high yielding cows obtain more nutrients for milk synthesis by digesting their diets more efficiently. To the contrary, one concern with higher feed intake is the potential for a depression in digestibility arising from higher rates of digesta passage through the gastrointestinal tract (Tyrrell and Moe, 1975. Van Soest, 1994; NRC, 2001). However, the depression in digestibility is greater for some feeds than others, and when comparing dry and lactating cows (Bines, Broster, Sutton, Broster, Napper, Smith and Siviter, 1988). The later observation suggests a physiological effect of lactation on digestion, in addition to an effect of intake level per se. That said, across a wide range of grass silage-based ration intakes in dry and lactating cattle, the ration digestible energy (DE) concentration (i.e. digestibility) was reduced proportionally by 0.025 with each increase in intake as a multiple of maintenance (Yan, Agnew and Gordon, 2002). The effect on ME concentration was lower (0.0168) because fractional losses of methane and urine energy were lower, which may reflect increased rate of passage and fractional retention of absorbed nitrogen, respectively. This reduced digestibility with greater intake appears to be a direct effect of intake level and not genetic differences between animals. In direct comparisons of low- and high-yielding genetic lines of cattle, at relatively similar levels of dry matter intake, there is no evidence of a difference in the fractional recovery of DE from intake energy or ME from DE (Belyea and Adams, 1990; Gordon *et al.*, 1995). Similarly, increases in milk yield of cows treatment with growth hormone is not accompanied by changes in ration digestibility, although fractional losses of methane were increased (Tyrrell, Brown, Reynolds, Haaland, Bauman, Peel and Steinhour, 1998).

Energetic efficiency

As milk yield increases are the nutrients supplied for milk production used more efficiently? There are surprisingly few comparisons of the efficiency of dietary nutrient use for milk production across breeds or strains of cattle. However, in terms of net energy for lactation (NE_l; milk energy corrected for body tissue energy gain or loss, excess N absorption and gestation), the incremental response to increasing ME is similar in lactating Holstein and beef cattle when expressed on a metabolic body weight (live weight$^{.75}$) basis (Reynolds and Tyrrell, 2000). The difference in milk yield capacity between the breeds alters the extent to which ME is partitioned towards milk energy and away from body tissue, and thus the amount of 'surplus' energy available for body fat synthesis, not the overall efficiency of ME use for net anabolic purposes. Similarly, comparisons of low- and high-yielding genetic lines of dairy cows found no differences in the efficiency of ME use for milk energy (Belyea and Adams, 1990; Gordon *et al.*, 1995). In terms of maintenance requirement, the high yielding cow is more efficient as maintenance cost per unit milk is diluted (Tyrrell *et al.*, 1998). However, recent data from the UK suggests that maintenance energy requirement is higher in modern dairy cows, perhaps as a consequence of differences in body composition (protein composition) or dietary influences which affect visceral tissue mass (Agnew and Yan, 2000; Kebreab, France, Agnew, Yan, Dhanoa, Dijkstra, Beever and Reynolds, 2003).

Body energy loss and partitioning

The effect of high milk yield on energy partition is exemplified by the loss of body energy in early lactation, a hallmark of the rising phase of lactation in modern dairy cows, when increases in milk energy output outpace increases in ME inputs, with consequent mobilization of body fat 'reserves' to balance the deficit. The extent of the loss varies with the magnitude and rate of increase of milk yield compared to ME intake, thus can be exacerbated if metabolic disease or management 'stumbles' impair intake. As total milk yield is proportional to peak milk yield, higher yielding cows have higher peak yields, and thus are presumed to be subject to more extensive body energy loss in early lactation. Lorna, the famous cow whose energy metabolism was measured whilst producing 49 kg of milk per day in 1964 (Flatt *et al.*, 1965 and 1969), exemplifies the cow who sacrifices body energy to support milk yield in early lactation. Lorna lost an average of 82 MJ/d of body tissue energy in early lactation, and 143 kg of live weight, but in late lactation she replenished her body energy at a rate of 77 MJ/d, and regained 135 kg of live weight. These results suggested to many that Lorna's excessive energy loss and gain represented a biological requirement for high milk yield, with energy 'banked' as body fat in late lactation to meet payments required in early lactation. This led to management strategies which emphasized body condition gain in late lactation, an approach justified in part by the finding that the efficiency of ME use for tissue energy gain is greater during lactation than in the dry period (Moe, Tyrrell and Flatt, 1971).

Do modern dairy cows loose more body energy than their predecessors under similar environmental conditions? In a recent calorimetry study (Hattan, Beever, Cammell and Sutton, 2001; Table 1), 6 cows in early lactation produced 50 kg of milk, consumed 25 kg of DM and lost 14 MJ of tissue energy daily, during the same period of lactation, Lorna and 11 of her herd mates produced an average of 29 kg of milk, consumed 12 kg of DM and lost 29 MJ of tissue energy daily (Flatt *et al.*, 1969). This comparison is obviously confounded in time and by differences in ration and other management influences, but emphasizes that the increase in milk yield of modern dairy cows has been accompanied by increased feed intake capacity. A more controlled comparison has been made using production data from 2 genetic lines of cattle (Crooker *et al.*, 2001), a control group maintained using genetics comparable to the breed average in 1964, and a selected line obtained using the 4 bulls ranked highest annually for production traits in the US (see Hansen, 2000). At the time of the study the average milk yields for the 2 lines differed by 4500 kg per 305 d lactation. The control cows were smaller and consumed less DMI, in both gestation and lactation. Estimated ME intake and milk energy output were greater for the selected line, but tissue energy balance did not differ between the 2 lines, reaching the same nadir of -64 MJ/d at 7 d postpartum and then becoming more positive, but remaining negative in both lines until 60 days in milk (Crooker *et al.*, 2001). Although cows from both lines lost large amounts of body energy in the first days of lactation, the data show that in cows managed to achieve adequate ME intakes, higher milk yields of modern dairy cows do not require more tissue energy and body condition than occurs in lower yielding dairy cows. Obviously, as milk yield increases the management challenge of meeting their dietary nutrient needs becomes greater. This implies that increases in milk yield achieved through genetics challenge, and thus improve, management systems such that genetics and nutrition improve in concert.

However, not all high yielding cows are capable of achieving adequate ration energy intake, especially under extensive or grass-based management systems (Veerkamp, Simm and Oldham, 1995; Buckley *et al.*, 2000; Harris and Kolver, 2001). In this case, the physiological drive to partition ME towards milk occurs at the expense of body tissue energy, as occurred in Lorna. In 3 studies where cows differing in their genetic potential for milk yield were managed using grazing or grass-silage based-rations, the cows selected for higher milk yield had lower body condition scores (Table 2). In the study reporting initial and final condition score (Gordon *et al.*, 1995), cows with the highest genetic merit ended the 150 day trial with slightly lower body condition than when the trial began, whilst those of medium or low genetic merit gained body condition (Table 2). This effect of genetics on body condition was exacerbated when concentrate allowance was restricted (Table 2; Veerkamp, Simm and Oldham, 1995). The effects of bovine growth hormone treatment provide a paradigm for the effects of genetic selection for greater milk yield on energy partition. Higher yielding cows typically have higher circulating levels of growth hormone, and lower levels of insulin, and growth hormone levels are lower in early lactation when the hormonal drive for milk synthesis is greatest. In the short term, growth hormone treatment increases milk energy output at the expense of body tissue energy (Tyrrell *et al.*, 1988). However, given the opportunity, ration intake of cows treated with growth hormone increases to provide adequate ME for the increase in milk energy yield, and ultimately the replenishment of the additional tissue energy lost (Bauman, 1992).

Table 1. Comparison of feed dry matter intake, milk yield and energy metabolism measured in high yielding dairy cows in 1964 and 1999.

	Early lactation		*Mid-lactation*	
	1964[1]	*1999*[2]	*1964*	*1999*
Dry matter intake, kg/d	12.0	24.7	13.2	24.4
Milk yield, kg/d	29.4	49.7	19.5	41.8
Energy balance, MJ/d				
Metabolisable energy (ME)	146	286	156	291
Heat energy	97	162	100	160
Milk energy	78	138	51	121
Tissue energy	-29	-14	5	10

[1]Flatt *et al.*, 1969. Average measurements from 12 cows at 4 to 15 (mean 8, early lactation) and 17 to 32 (mean 24, mid-lactation) weeks postpartum.
[2]Hattan *et al.*, 2001. Average measurements from 6 cows at 6 and 12 (early lactation) and 18 and 24 (mid-lactation) weeks postpartum.

Table 2. Effect of selection for milk yield on average dry matter intake (DMI; kg/d), milk yield (kg/d), milk fat (g/kg), body condition score (BCS; 5 point scale) and body weight (BWT; kg) in cows fed grass silage or grazing grass in the UK or Ireland.

	DIM[1]	*DMI*	*Milk yield*	*Milk fat*	*BCS*[2]	*BCS Δ*[3]	*BWT*[4]
Gordon *et al.*, 1995							
Low	11-160	19.0	29.0	36.9	3.22	0.52	528
Medium	11-160	19.4	30.6	39.7	3.34	0.54	551
High	11-160	20.2	37.2	37.8	2.55	-0.18	631
Veerkamp, Simm and Oldham, 1995							
High concentrate							
Control	1-182	17.6	27.5	41.2	2.54	-	602
Select	1-182	18.3	32.0	40.8	2.40	-	611
Low concentrate							
Control	1-182	15.2	22.7	44.8	2.51	-	594
Select	1-182	15.7	26.3	44.9	2.28	-	596
Buckley *et al.*, 2000							
Grazing							
Low	56-265	17.5	25.0	39.2	2.99	-	554
High	56-265	18.5	28.2	36.7	2.54	-	553
Grass silage							
Low	28	17.9	35.9	40.4	3.40	-	603
High	28	18.2	39.6	38.6	2.84	-	601

[1]Days in milk.
[2]Final or average body condition score.
[3]Body condition score change from calving to end of study.
[4]Initial or average body weight.

Consequences of greater milk yield

What are the consequences of high yield for the dairy cow? Under conditions of limited dietary energy input, as occurs with grazing or many grass silage-based rations, higher yielding cows typically finish lactation with less body condition (Buckley *et al.*, 2000; Harris and Kolver, 2001; Veerkamp, Simm and Oldham, 1995; Gordon *et al.*, 1995). This may reflect a limitation of surplus energy after the nadir of tissue energy loss in early lactation, and not necessarily a greater body energy loss in early lactation per se. Perhaps the most documented change associated with increased milk yield potential has been a decline in fertility (e.g. Lucy, 2001). A summary of 6 studies comparing the performance of NA and New Zealand (NZ) Holstein cows within intensively managed grazing systems in NZ concluded that NA cows produced more milk and milk protein, but had lower fertility and body condition (Harris and Kolver, 2001). The NA cows were less likely to survive to later lactations, but this was largely due to reduced fertility and the strict need for yearly calving intervals.

Causes for the global decline in fertility of higher yielding cows are uncertain. The association between 'high' milk yield (relative to breed averages) and fertility is not a modern phenomenon; it was noted as early as 1929 (Hansen, 2000). Excessive body energy loss in early lactation delays the return of oestrus, and has been associated with a reduced first service conception rate, thus the decline in fertility of modern dairy cows is often blamed on excessive body energy loss in early lactation (Staples, Thatcher and Clark, 1990; Lucy, 2001). Again, excessive tissue energy loss in early lactation is not a requirement for high milk yield, or restricted to high yielding cows. In one study, cows were grouped by reproductive status and the group with the highest incidence of anestrus had the greatest calculated tissue energy loss in the first 2 weeks of lactation, but were also the lowest yielding cows in the study (Staples, Thatcher and Clark, 1990). In the US, the reduction in fertility observed nationally is not restricted to higher yielding herds, which often have better fertility due to better management, and the decline in fertility may not be due to greater body energy loss *per se*, but may be due to other genetic or environmental changes (Lucy, 2001; Harris and Kolver, 2001). A simple explanation proposed is that a shortage of glucose and other energy yielding metabolites demanded by the mammary gland impairs reproductive functions of the ovary or other body tissues (McClure, 1994).

Do modern dairy cows live shorter lives? Although not a true measure of longevity, the breeding value for productive life of US Holsteins dropped from 27 months in 1960 to 24 months in the mid-1990s, but has since increased to 26 months (Figure 2). Meanwhile, the breeding value for milk yield has doubled. The USDA estimate of productive life (www.aipl.arsusda.gov) assumes a 10 month lactation, which is no longer the norm in many high yielding herds with extended lactations, and shifts in cow age and 'longevity' also reflect national culling and replacement activity, which is driven by economic and policy pressure. Whilst herd turnover has increased since 1960, cows staying in the herd stay longer, in part due to longer lactations. Metabolically, increases in intake and milk yield in early lactation require greater blood flow, oxidative metabolism and associated heat production to digest, absorb, deliver and use nutrients for milk synthesis and remove metabolic end-products, thus heart rate and cardiac output are increased. In a recent study in transition dairy cows, blood flow and oxygen consumption by the digestive tract and liver more than doubled after calving, with the majority of the increase occurring in the first 11 days of lactation, presumably as a consequence of increased intake, as well as glucose synthesis and oxidative metabolism by the liver (Reynolds, Aikman, Lupoli, Humphries and Beever, 2003). Intuitively, this increase in metabolic workload may have consequences for immune function, health and welfare of the cow, but apart from mastitis and lameness, where, as for fertility, management influences are critical, supportive evidence is scarce (Lucy, 2001; Pryce, Veerkamp, Thompson, Hill and Simm, 1997). Positive genetic correlations between milk yield and mastitis, milk fever and lameness have been reported (Pryce *et al.*, 1997). In a meta-analysis of data from commercial herds treated with bovine growth hormone, treatment beginning after peak lactation had no effect on fertility or the incidence of mastitis, but was also associated with an increase in the incidence of foot disorders (Collier, Byatt, Denham, Eppard, Fabellar, Hintz, McGrath, McLaughlin, Shearer, Veenhuizen and Vicini, 2001). These increases in foot disorders in higher yielding cows have been attributed to greater intakes of fermentable carbohydrates, and rumen acid load, resulting from diet formulations to increase ration ME density, thus also reflect an interaction between level of milk yield and management practice.

Changing the lactation curve

There is a consistent relationship between peak milk and total yield, thus high peak yields are thought to be required for high milk yield (Clark and Davis, 1980). As average milk yield increases, peak yield increases, but persistency declines (Chase, 1993). As greater peak yields stress the need for maximal ME intake in early lactation, there is currently interest in the feasibility of manipulating the shape of the lactation curve such that high milk yield is achieved with lower peak yields, as proposed by Ferris, Mao and Anderson (1985). The concept is based on a shift in production from early to later lactation via a slower rise to peak, and a more persistent, flatter lactation after peak yield is reached. This may be achieved through genetic selection, as lactation persistency is a heritable trait, or perhaps nutritional management. However, the biological basis of the lactation 'curve' (changes in cell number and capacity) may make it difficult to delay or reduce peak milk yield without sacrificing total yield. A previous study found selection for persistency reduced peak, and thus total, milk yield (Ferris, Mao and Anderson, 1985), but Wood's equation was used to describe lactation profile, which forces a relationship between peak yield and persistency. The potential benefits of these changes in lactation curve characteristics for cow fertility and health merit further investigation.

Conclusions

So how has the high yielding cow changed in the last 40 years? Compared to Lorna and her cohorts, she is certainly bigger, more angular, and capable of greater feed consumption. Through progress in genetics and management, today's high yielding cows are better equipped to produce large amounts of milk with less loss in body tissue than Lorna. Along the way there has been a decline in fertility, and a consequent overall reduction in productive life, especially in low input pasture-based management systems with strict calving intervals. In higher input systems, allowing cows to express their full potential for nutrient intake and milk synthesis, high yielding cows that reproduce produce more milk for longer lactations. Over the last 50 years, increases in the genetic potential for milk yield have challenged cow management practice. As when Friesians replaced Shorthorns, and then Holsteins replaced Friesians, genetic improvement requires improvements in nutritional and reproductive management, and the bar continues to rise.

References

Agnew, R. E. and Yan, T. (2000) Impact of recent research on energy feeding systems for dairy cattle. *Livestock Production Science*, **66**, 197-215.

Bauman, D.E. (1992) Bovine somatotropin: review of an emerging animal technology. *Journal of Dairy Science*, **75**, 3432-3451.

Belyea, R.L. and Adams, M.W. (1990) Energy and nitrogen utilization of high versus low producing dairy cows. *Journal of Dairy Science*, **73**, 1023-1030.

Bines, J.A., Broster, W.H., Sutton, J.D., Broster, V.J., Napper, D.J., Smith, T. and Siviter, J.W. (1988) Effect of amount consumed and diet composition on the apparent digestibility of feed in cattle and sheep. *Journal of Agricultural Science, Cambridge*, **110**, 249-259.

Buckley, F., Dillon, P., Rath, M. and Veerkamp, R. F. (2000) The relationship between genetic merit for yield and live weight, condition score, and energy balance of spring calving Holstein Friesian dairy cows on grass based systems of milk production. *Journal of Dairy Science*, **83**, 1878-1886.

Chase, L. E. (1993) Developing nutrition programs for high producing dairy herds. *Journal of Dairy Science*, **76**, 3287-3293.

Clark, J.H. and Davis, C.L. (1980) Some aspects of feeding high producing dairy cows. *Journal of Dairy Science*, **63**, 873-885.

Collier, R.J., Byatt, J.C., Denham, S.C., Eppard, P.J., Fabellar, A.C., Hintz, R.L., McGrath, M.F., McLaughlin, C.L., Shearer, J.K., Veenhuizen, J.J. and Vicini, J.L. (2001) Effects of sustained release bovine somatotropin (Sometribove) on animal health in commercial dairy herds. *Journal of Dairy Science*, **84**, 1098-1108.

Crooker, B.A., Weber, W.J., Ma, L.S. and Lucy, M.C. (2001) Effect of energy balance and selection for milk yield on the somatotropic axis of the lactating Holstein cow: endocrine profiles and hepatic gene expression. *In Proceedings of the 15th Symposium on Energy Metabolism in Animals, Energy Metabolism in Animals,* pp. 345-348. Edited by A. Chwalibog and K. Jakobsen. Wageningen Pers, Wageningen, The Netherlands.

Ferris, T. A., Mao, I. L., and Anderson, C. R. (1985) Selection for lactation curve and milk yield in dairy cattle. *Journal of Dairy Science*, **68**, 1438-1448.

Flatt, W.P., Moe, P.W., Munson, A.W. and Cooper, T. (1969) Energy utilization by high producing dairy cows. II. Summary of energy balance experiments with lactating Holstein cows. *In Energy Metabolism of Farm Animals,* pp. 235 - 249. Edited by K.L. Blaxter, J. Kielanowski and G. Thorbeck. Oriel Press, Newcastle-upon-Tyne, UK.

Flatt, W.P., Moore, L.A., Hooven, N.W., and R.D. Plowman. (1965) Energy metabolism studies with a high producing lactating dairy cow. *Journal of Dairy Science,* **48**, 797-798.

Gordon, F.J., Patterson, D.C., Yan, T., Porter, M.G., Mayne, C.S. and Unsworth, E.F. (1995) The influence of genetic index for milk production on the response to complete diet feeding and the utilization of energy and nitrogen. *Animal Science,* **61**, 199-210.

Hansen, L. B. (2000) Consequences of selection for milk yield from a geneticist's point of view. *Journal of Dairy Science,* **83**, 1145-1150.

Harris, B.L. and Kolver, E.S. (2001) Review of Holsteinization on intensive pastoral dairy farming in New Zealand. *Journal of Dairy Science,* **84** (Electronic Supplement): E56-E61.

Hattan, A.J., Beever, D.E., Cammell, S.B. and Sutton, J.D. (2001) Energy metabolism in high yielding dairy cows during early lactation. *In Proceedings of the 15th Symposium on Energy Metabolism in Animals, Energy Metabolism in Animals,* pp. 325-328. Edited by A. Chwalibog, and K. Jakobsen. Wageningen Pers, Wageningen, The Netherlands.

Kebreab, E., France, J., Agnew, R.E., Yan, T., Dhanoa, M.S., Dijkstra, J., Beever, D.E. and Reynolds, C.K. (2003) Alternatives to linear analysis of energy balance data from lactating dairy cows. *Journal of Dairy Science*, **86**, 2904-2913.

Lucy, M.C. (2001) Reproductive loss in high-producing dairy cattle: Where will it end? *Journal of Dairy Science,* **84**, 277-1293.

McClure, T.J. (1994) *Nutritional and Metabolic Infertility in the Cow.* CABI International, Wallingford, UK.

Moe, P.W., Tyrrell, H.F. and Flatt, W.P. (1971) Energetics of body tissue mobilisation. *Journal of Dairy Science,* **54**, 548-553.

NRC. (2001) *Nutrient Requirements of Dairy Cattle (7th Edition).* National Academy Press, Washington, DC.

Pryce, J.E., Veerkamp, R.F., Thompson, R., Hill, W.G., and Simm, G. (1997) Genetic aspects of common health disorders and measures of fertility in Holstein Friesian dairy cattle. *Animal Science*, 65, 353-360.

Reynolds, C.K. and Tyrrell, H.F. (2000) Energy metabolism in lactating beef heifers. *Journal of Animal Science*, 78, 2696-2705.

Reynolds, C.K., Aikman, P.C., Lupoli, B., Humphries, D.J., and Beever, D.E. (2003) Splanchnic metabolism of dairy cows during the transition from late gestation through early lactation. *Journal of Dairy Science*, 86, 1201-1217.

Staples, C.R., Thatcher, W.W., and Clark, J.H. (1990) Relationship between ovarian activity and energy status during the early postpartum period of high producing dairy cows. *Journal of Dairy Science*, 73, 938-947.

Tyrrell, H.F., Brown, A.C.G., Reynolds, P.J., Haaland, G.L., Bauman, D.E., Peel, C.J. and Steinhour, W.D. (1988) Effect of bovine somatotropin on metabolism of lactating dairy cows: energy and nitrogen utilization as determined by respiration calorimetry. *Journal of Nutrition*, 118, 1024-1030.

Tyrrell, H.F. and Moe, P.W. (1975) Effect of intake on digestive efficiency. *Journal of Dairy Science*, 58, 1151 – 1163.

Van Soest, P.J. (1994) *Nutritional Ecology of the Ruminant*. O & B Books, Inc., Corvallis, Oregon, USA.

Yan, T., Agnew, R.E. and Gordon, F. J. (2002) The combined effects of animal species (sheep *versus* cattle) and level of feeding on digestible and metabolizable energy concentrations of grass-based diets of cattle. *Animal Science*, 75, 141-151.

Veerkamp, R.F., Simm, G., and Oldham, J.D. (1995) Genotype by environment interactions: experience from Langhill. *In Breeding and Feeding the High Genetic Merit Dairy Cow*, pp. 59-66. Edited by T.J. Lawrence, F.J. Gordon and A. Carson. Occasional Publication No. 19, British Society of Animal Science.

4

LONGEVITY

David N. Logue[1], Alistair W. Stott[2], John Santarossa[3], George J. Gunn[4] and Jill E. Offer[1]
SAC Veterinary Services (Ayr[1] & Inverness[4]), Land Economy Group (Ayr[3] & Aberdeen[2]) SAC, West Mains Road Edinburgh, UK

Introduction

Investigations of culling and particularly involuntary culling ("functional" longevity) have often used different criteria on herds of varying size in different regions and with divergent average milk outputs (Young, Waddington, Sales, Bradley and Spooner, 1983; Esslemont and Kossaibati, 1997; Forbes, Gayton and McGeogh, 1999; Whitaker Kelly and Smith, 2000; Figure 1). Thus the evidence of increasing or decreasing culling for any particular entity is uncertain. However it can be deduced that generally UK dairy herds cull 25% of their cattle, the majority of which are involuntary culls and that infertility, mastitis and lameness are the main reasons for the culling.

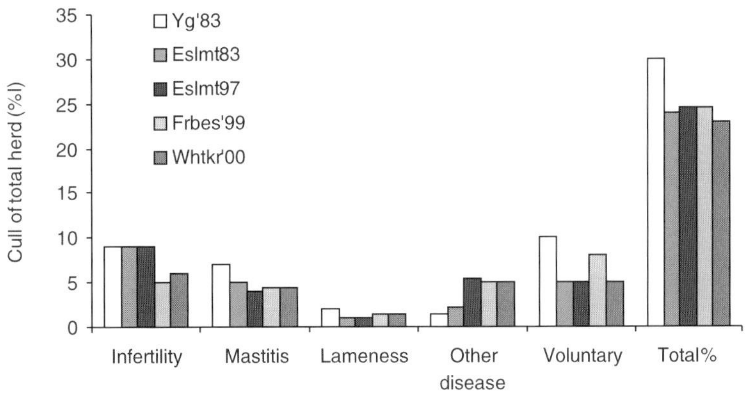

Figure 1 Summary of some culling information in UK dairy herds

These conditions have been the subject of considerable research for many years. As our understanding of the risk factors for them has grown, so also has the realisation that culling and thus longevity is best considered as an economic decision (Stott, 1994; Veerkamp, Hill, Stott, Brotherstone and Simm, 1994). The need to involve economics in any discussion of dairy cattle management has been strengthened recently by the Farm Animal Welfare Council who identified these conditions as the main determinants of welfare in the dairy cow (Anon, 1997). They associated the need for their improved control with the growing demand for quality food products from UK agriculture rather than cheap food commodities (Harvey, 2001). It is therefore far from encouraging that despite all the technology transfer, the improved general management and facilities for dairy cows and undoubted advances in farmer education that, apart from mastitis, there seems to be little or no overall improvement in these conditions (Whitaker Kelly and Smith, 2000). Developments in the genetics and management of dairy cattle associated with increasing yield have been related to an increased prevalence in these conditions and so by inference culling and functional longevity (Pryce, Veerkamp, Thompson, Hill and Simm, 1998). Unfortunately, like culling, disease recording by farmers, and even researchers, is frequently inadequately defined, poorly controlled and highly variable and this has caused geneticists and their related co-workers considerable difficulties. We suggest that in the short and medium term a more focused farmer input into the day to day management of their cows is the best strategy for improving the longevity of their dairy cows and that by improving and standardising disease recording the necessary groundwork for genetic improvement can be laid.

Reproduction and Infertility

Biosecurity and the proper monitoring of disease in the dairy herd are generally inadequately addressed on most farms though this is improving thanks to farm assurance. It has taken a Foot-and-Mouth outbreak to remind farmers and government policy makers of the importance of these issues (Anon, 2002). Control of infectious infertility is an essential part of fertility control. Closed herds have been shown to have better fertility (number of births per 100 cows per year) than "open" ones with an economic value of approximately £25/cow (Schaik, Dijkhuizen, Benedictus, Barkema and Koole, 1998). Control of infectious infertility is an essential part of fertility control. Even now in some herds infectious agents such as *Leptospira hardjo,* IBR, BVD/MD, *Campylobacter fetus sp.,* and *Neospora caninum,* can be identified as the prime cause of the poor fertility. For a 50-cow herd with a 50 % death rate for persistently infected animals and a milk price of 18ppl the median annual loss due to BVD over a ten-year period was estimated to be over £10,000. For a 200 cow herd under the same assumptions, the median loss over a ten year period was estimated to be over £56,000 (Gunn, Stott, Humphry and Jones, 2000). Altogether these data suggest that both government and the industry need to examine the cost benefits of increased biosecurity in various types of livestock units more closely and develop their policies on a sound scientific and economic basis.

Fertility in the UK does appear to be falling (Royal, Darwash, Flint, Webb, Williams and Lamming, 2000). Modern breeding and management techniques have produced dairy cows with an ability to yield large amounts of milk at considerable expense to their body reserves and these factors have been linked with reduced fertility. Furthermore in some herds there seems to be a considerable proportion of late embryonic and early foetal losses. It is assumed that many of these are "physiological" rather than infectious but the underlying mechanisms are still being defined (Royal *et al.*, 2000; Sreenan, Diskin and Morris, 2001; O'Callaghan, Lozano, Fahey, Gath, Snijders and Boland, 2001; Butler, 2001; Thatcher, Binelli, Arnold, Mattos, Badinga, Moreira, Staples and Guzeloglu, 2001). As with culling, any review of information from the field is fraught with difficulties of interpretation. Figure 2 attempts to summarise some of the present field evidence for a fall in fertility with time in the UK and confirms that a regular review of consistent, reliable large-scale field data would be very useful in assuring us of the magnitude of this change. In addition there have been many changes in fertility management over this time period and some of these may well also have had detrimental effects on overall herd fertility. These various interpretational problems have been amply described for many years (Boyd and Reed, 1961a,b;Watson, Jones and Saunders,1987; Lucey and Croker, 2001).

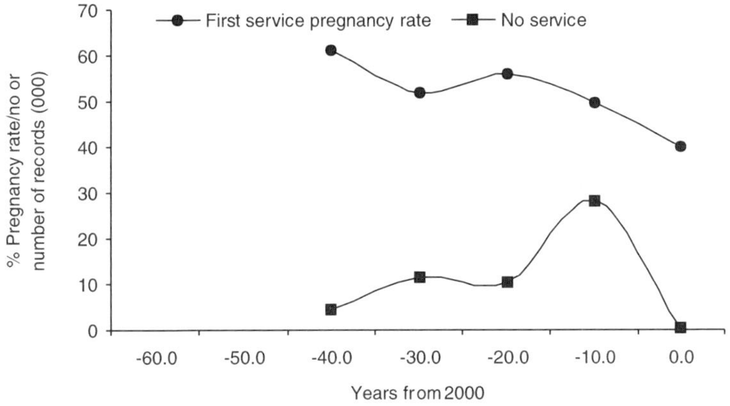

Figure 2
A summary of the effect of time on "pregnancy rate" to first service based on data derived from UK dairy herds.

Recent studies suggest that, while there is a limit to the extent that one can ask the cow to "milk off her back" without problems, for the majority of UK dairy farmers this is not yet a major issue. (Webb, Garnsworthy, Gong, Robinson and Wathes, 1999; Webb, Garnsworthy, Gong, Gutterrez, Logue, Crawshaw and Robinson, 1997; Knight, Beever and Sorensen, 1999). Thus, although Webb *et al.* (1997) reported that that high genetic merit cows take some 8 days longer to first ovulation post-calving than control cows and that nutrition can affect follicular development, some farms seem to be able to maintain fertility despite these difficulties (Kossaibati and Esslemont, 1997). Similar findings regarding the effect of genetics, season and nutrition on fertility have been variously reported (Ryan and Mee, 1994; O'Farrell, 1998; Logue, Berry, Offer, Chaplin, Crawshaw, Leach, Ball and Bax, 1999; Sreenan, Diskin and Morris, 2001; O'Callaghan *et al.*, 2001; Lucey and Crooker, 2001; Lindhe and Philipsson, 2001). Together these data introduce the concern that those dairy farmers striving to obtain maximum yield from forage-fed high genetic merit cows and also maintain a tight calving pattern, may well find this fertility effect a considerable limitation on productivity (Cromie, Gordon, Kelleher and Rath, 1998).

Irrespective of these factors it is crucial that farmers concentrate on maintaining high calving rates to service (especially first service, the most reliable estimate of this). This means the use of high fertility semen, experienced inseminators, the limitation of specific and non-specific disease associated with infertility and careful overall management (including nutrition) of the cows. It is well documented that different bulls both in natural service and in AI have different fertility rates (Logue and Isbister 1992). Presently UK farmers are not given good information about this partly for statistical reasons and partly because of commercial confidentiality. Recently, an economic model herd involving fertility factors alongside other farm factors has been developed by Santarossa and Stott (pers. comm.) from an earlier prototype (Stott, Veerkamp and Wassell, 1999). This shows that a reduction in bull fertility of as little as 0.05 (0.5 to 0.45) has a cost of the order of £10 per cow in the herd assuming all cows are mated to that bull (see Figure 3a). This finding highlights the urgent need for a more detailed economic examination of this and other related factors such as the balance between the generally lower calving rates with sexed semen, the speed of replacement production and genetic gain.

Accurate (correctly presented) and efficient (identified) oestrous detection is essential for good fertility when AI is used. All herd records suggest that, while most farmers are quite accurate at identifying oestrous cows (~95%), efficiency is more difficult (~80% is a good figure). Loss of efficiency is particularly apparent at the end of the breeding period when there are few cycling cows. Finally there is concern that oestrus expression is also subdued in the modern high yielding cow (Roche J. pers com 2003). The Santarossa & Stott model illustrates the importance of the link between oestrous detection efficiency (ODe) pregnancy rate and culling rate (Figure 3b). It also shows, not surprisingly, that it is costly to have a high ODe (implying large costly labour inputs) if the pregnancy rate is poor, say at much below 0.4 (see Figure 3a). Note also the law of diminishing returns at high pregnancy and oestrous detection rates.

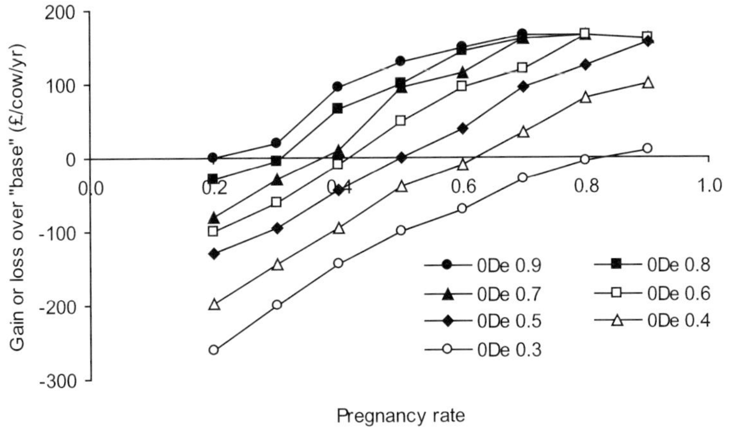

Figure 3a. The effect of pregnancy rate and oestrous detection efficiency (ODe) on income/cow/yr from Santarossa & Stott's Economic Model.

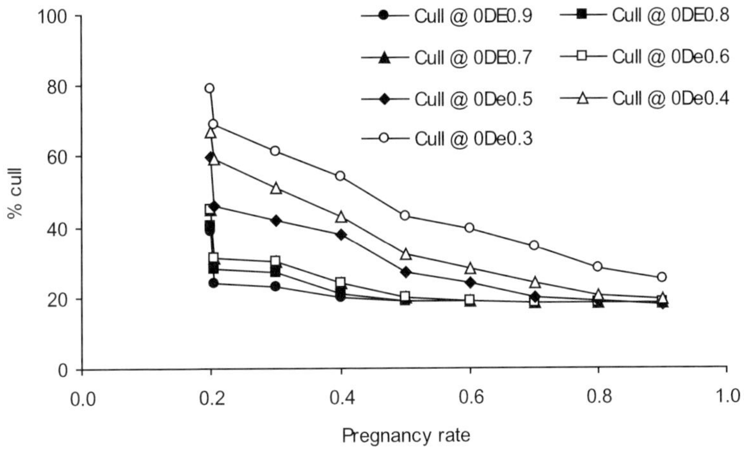

Figure 3b. The effect of pregnancy rate to all services and oestrous detection efficiency (ODe) on culling from Santarossa & Stott's Economic Model.

In summary farms should aim to use the best inseminator and high fertility bulls matching the intensity of oestrous detection to the level of fertility achieved. They should ensure adequate cow comfort and nutrition, keep a closed herd with good herd biosecurity, keep the cattle in small consistent groups, if possible matched by size, maintain and use records and finally but importantly utilise their veterinarians cost-effectively within a properly developed farm health plan. This does not mean cheaply! Once the breeding season is started it is very difficult to change matters so it is best to try to get things correct before breeding starts.

Mastitis and SCC control

Mastitis is of obvious concern to the farmer as it causes pain and directly affects milk output and quality (especially the bulk tank somatic cell counts or BTSCC) (Fitzpatrick, Young, Eckersall, Logue, Knight and Nolan, 1998; Eshraghi, Zeitlin, Fitzpatrick, Ternent and Logue,

1999). Webster (1995) raised the possibility that increasing stress might impair the immune system and as a consequence there might be an increase in the prevalence of mastitis (or indeed other diseases). In one instance in the Scottish Executive (SEERAD) funded Metabolic Stress Study there did appear to be an immune suppression in high genetic merit cows on a low input system compared to those on a high output system (Sinclair, Nielsen, Oldham and Reid, 1999). However in another there was none (Sinclair *unpublished information* 1998 see Logue *et al.*, 1999). This is an area needing more study.

It is easiest to consider mastitis as either clinical or subclinical, but this is a simplification: they are two ends of a spectrum. However in the past decade EU pressures on milk quality have led to a substantial reduction in subclinical mastitis and herd bulk tank SCC figures with UK national BTSCC figures having fallen by around 100,000. This improvement has been built around the application three basic principles of disease control, limiting the level of infection in the herd, suppressing the transfer of infection between cows and reducing any predisposing factors. However, recently national BTSCC figures have been rising. This is partly because, with lower milk prices, many herds have reached a position where they feel it is not economically worthwhile to push for the top SCC premium milk price at the expense of other economic factors. Thanks to another SAC model we have evidence that, unless they can maintain a low level of subclinical infection in the herd, this is quite a wise decision (Stott, Gunn, Humphry, Chase-Topping, Jones, Berry, Richardson and Logue, 2000).

While there are many bacteria that cause mastitis, reviews show that really only 6 are major pathogens and one of these *Arcanobacterium pyogenes* is most associated with summer or dry cow mastitis. The others (see Figure 4) can be arbitarily divided into "environmental" and "parlour" organisms. The environmental organisms, such as *Escherichia coli* and *Streptococcus uberis,* are usually more associated with clinical mastitis and therefore the presentation of single milk samples to the Veterinary Investigation Centre (VIC). However in some cases it would seem *S uberis* can also cause subclinical problems. The parlour organisms, most particularly *Staphylococcus aureus,* the most common and least amenable pathogen to treatment (Larsen, Sloth, Elsberg, Enevoldsen, Pedersen, Eriksen, Aarestrup and Jensen, 2000), can and do cause clinical mastitis. However they are quite frequently associated with subclinical mastitis i.e. multiple submission samples to the VIC taken after a herd SCC investigation as opposed to single samples for a clinical problem.

Thus for a herd with a significant *S. aureus* infection an economic balance needs to be struck between the level of infection, treatment and culling for SCC (to reduce that level of infection) and the overall management inputs. These include methods of limiting infection transfer between cows (Yalcin, Stott, Logue, and Gunn, 1999; Stott *et al.*, 2000). In essence a balance needs to be struck between mastitis control inputs and output from the herd (Yalcin *et al.*, 1999). This approach is even more crucial for organic farmers where control of the level of infection is limited by restrictions on antibiotic treatment and the adoption of treatments less likely to cure or limit the problem (Knight, Fitzpatrick, Logue, Platt, Robertson and Ternent, 2000). In many instances culling of intractable cases is the best method for reducing infection.

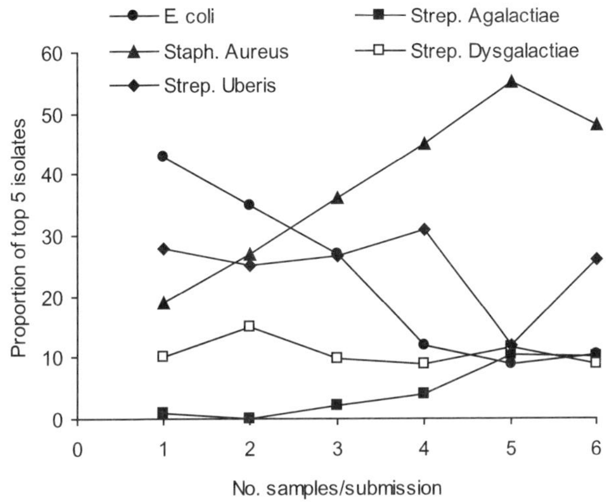

Figure 4. The effect of number of milk samples per submission on the organism isolated (SAC VIDA data 2001).

Table 1. "Equilibrium" BTSCC for Average (6,800 l/cow/year) yield herds in face of economic penalties of subclinical mastitis for yield output and milk price. These represent long-run targets for the herd and individual cow respectively using the model of Stott *et al.* (2000).

	BTSCC "Threshold" figures			
Level of infection in herd	*Before any SCC penalties etc*	*After culling effect of SCC (yield loss and milk price)*	*Reduction in BTSCC caused by considering subclinical mastitis*	*Difference in culling (for SCC) from control*
Control (Low)	149	128	21	0
Intermediate	213	167	46	2%
Infected	318	191	127	5%

The effect of this culling is quite subtle with cows at different lactations and with different individual SCCs having different culling criteria within each type of herd. This is best illustrated by using the model (Stott, Jones, Gunn, Chase-Topping, Humphry, Richardson and Logue, 2002) to compare a more severely affected infected herd with one with a low level of infection – so-called control. Figure 5 shows that the effect is for the infected herd to cull more through out the herd but particularly heavily in the 4th and 5th lactations (proportionately by a factor of 3).

In summary, economics demand that farmers must now be much more aware of the clinical and subclinical mastitis status of their herds. Information is the key. They must use individual cow SCC figures alongside bacteriological investigations of both clinical and subclinical infections to determine the extent of infection and types of organism acting in the herd. This information allows the farmer and his veterinarian to decide on priorities and the best balance between control inputs, their cost and potential reward (see Table 2). Mastitis and BTSCC control require both care and long-term planning.

Figure 5. The effect of infection on culling against high SCC cows within either "Control" (or so-called "Uninfected herd") and "Infected herd" according to the model of Stott *et al.* (2000).

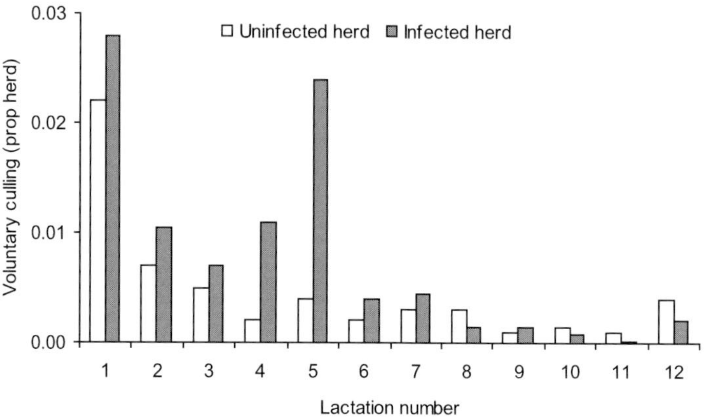

Lameness

Lameness has a considerable economic effect upon the dairy herd. Not only is there milk loss from treatment and reduced production but most importantly it is also associated with reduced fertility (Collick, Ward and Dobson, 1989; Hernandez, Shearer and Webb, 2001). Estimates of lameness incidence vary with study but generally it is considerably more common than is often recorded in farmer records (Wells, Trent, Marsh and Robinson, 1993; Clarkson, Downham, Faull, Hughes, Manson, Merrit, Murray, Russell, Suthrest and Ward, 1996; Whay, Main, Green, and Webster, 2002). In a recent MDC Link Project in Scotland farmers underestimated lameness prevalence by more 50% (Mason, Bagnall, Offer, Lyon, Logue and Roberts, 2003 unpublished). An estimate of increase in calving interval caused by different lameness conditions (simplified into claw horn lesions and digital/interdigital lesions) based on the literature is shown in Table 3.

Table 3. Range of literature estimates of the effect of lameness on calving interval of affected cows and "summary" estimate

Condition	*Range of effect on calving interval (days)*	*"Summary" estimate of increase*
Claw horn lesion	19 to 70	20
Digital/interdigital lesion	0 to 20	5

Table 2. On farm approaches to the prevention and control of mastitis.

Reason for strategy	*Five Point Plan*	*Additional strategies*
Reduce level of infection	Use dry cow therapy Treat clinical cases immediately Treat selected subclinical cases Cull problem cows (Record)	1. Improve RECORDING of clinical cases & sample a proportion for bacteriology (at least 10/year) 2. Use ICSCC to select problem cows and: a. Determine major organisms (bacteriology on at least 10 samples) b. Target treatment/dry cow therapy (sensitivity etc) c. If intractable mastitis target culling using above rationale d. Ensure good teat condition limit sores etc.
Limit transfer	Use post milking teat dipping	1. Milk low ICSCC cows (heifers) first 2. If udders clean dry wipe with an individual paper towel (depends on "TBC") 3. Use a premilking teat dip at critical times
Limit predisposing factors	Regular milking machine maintenance (& test)	1. Assess machine critically (ACRs, liner replacement etc) 2. Evaluate housing and management to increase cow cleanliness 3. Make cows stand post-milking.

Using these estimates within the recent SAC economic model we compared a herd with a low incidence of these conditions to an "average" herd. The assumptions of incidence are largely based on the Liverpool survey (Clarkson *et al.,* 1996). The "average" herd had not only an increased overall culling rate compared to the "control" (by approximately 5%) but also a "financial penalty" of well in excess of £20/cow in the herd. Note that this ignores any other costs of the lesion such as treatment and discarded milk etc., which, for a sole ulcer, may amount to over £80 per affected cow (or approximately £10/cow in the herd) (Kossaibati and Esslemont, 1997). Furthermore using these figures this model is suggesting that for the average herd the economic weight of losses due to claw horn lesions considerably outweigh digital/ interdigital lesions. Thus these calculations suggest that focussing solely on digital dermatitis and ignoring claw horn conditions is misplaced especially when there is good information that action to produce clean dry underfoot housing conditions will limit the former considerably (Rodriguez-Lainz, Hird, Carpenter, and Read, 1996; Rodriguez-Lainz, Melendez-Retamal, Hird, Read and Walker, 1999).

Controlling claw horn lesions is more difficult as they appear to have a complex aetiology and pathogenesis. They develop from defects in the integrity of the claw horn, particularly from haemorrhages resulting from damage to the horn producing epithelium of the claw. Figure 6a from Le Fevre (2003) presents the modelled profile for the lesion score for the sole of all feet with time post-calving in 12 groups (or cohorts) of first calving heifers (8 to 30 per group) that were then housed in cubicles. White line lesions follow a different pattern and show an earlier peak post calving. Heifers were used because it is generally considered that, since the feet of these young cows are usually the least affected before calving, they are a more reliable indicator of response to risk factors than older animals that may have been affected by previous lameness and lesions Figure 6b).

Despite this complication older cows still show a similar if less well-defined pattern (Offer, McNulty and Logue, 1999). Indeed we are now aware that even heifers are subject to such influences (Offer, Fisher, Kempson and Logue, 2001; Offer, Leach, Brocklehurst and Logue, 2003).

The presence of these peaks between 2 to 4 month post partum agrees well with a number of estimates of peak lameness from the literature and with other similar lesion development studies (Livesey and Fleming, 1984; Peterse, Korver, Oldenbroek and Talmon, 1984; Huang, Shanks and McCoy, 1995; Bergsten and Herlin, 1995; Livesey, Harrington, Johnston, May and Metcalf, 1998; Webster, 2001). Taken together these results illustrate the importance of considering management before and around the calving period as well as the post –calving period in the main milking herd in any control strategy.

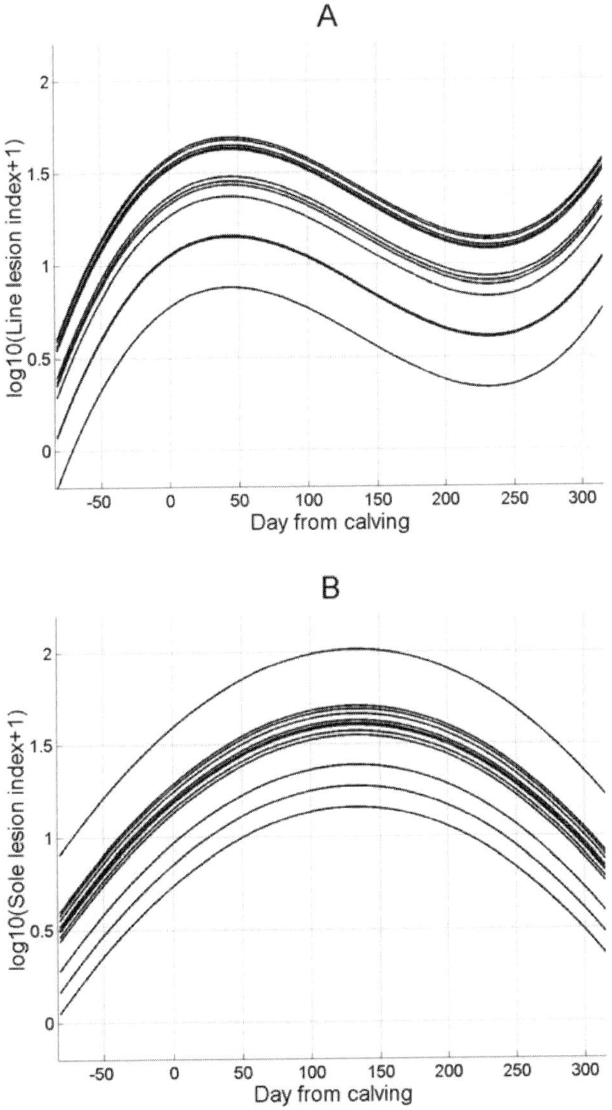

Figure 6a & b. Estimated fixed effect modelling of days from calving for combined datasets of first calving heifers in all SAC studies with image analysis of lesions by "white line" lesions (a) and "sole" lesions (b). Different lines are different SAC treatments and exposure groups. (Le Fevre, 2003)

Recently we have reviewed over 1000 papers on lameness in an attempt to further define good on-farm interventions (Hirst, Le Fevre, Logue, Offer, Chaplin, Murray, Ward and French, 2002). While we are now in a position to define each study within our systematic review in terms of the statistical strength this has, as yet, a limited application. This is because many different outcomes of "lameness" have been used and even something as simple as incidence of lameness has proved far from easy to relate between papers. Secondly the recording of explanatory and other variables has been equally difficult (Logue, 2002; Le Fevre, Hirst, French, Offer, Brocklehurst, Gibbs, Laven, Gettinby and Logue, 2002). This has meant the categorisation and simplification of the various studies to allow grouping the papers. For example of the papers studying lameness by housing type (cubicle or straw yard) giving verifiable data 13/19 (68%) showed a significant positive association between lameness and cubicle housing only, 2/19 papers suggested that cubicle housing reduced lameness while 4/19 were essentially neutral either because this was the case for their study or they did not use sufficient animals or herds. Thus, in our opinion, the summary that the "strength" of evidence of 68% for a cubicle housing system with its harder, rougher and less resilient flooring to be associated with more lameness than a straw yard is a useful guide for the farmer. However this approach is very simplistic. Different conditions may have different risk factors. Thus although Alban, Lawson and Agger (1995) found more lameness at grazing than when housed, they were only considering one specific condition, Foul-in-the-Foot. Similarly our approach does not attempt to weigh the different strengths of evidence of the various studies or their relative merits in terms of design and approach.

The exact reasons for the significant associations between herd size, average herd yield and lameness indicated by this review are open to debate. However there seems little doubt that the foot of the cow was not designed to be housed and to walk on concrete and functions best at grass (Faye and Lescourret, 1989; Whitaker Kelly and Smith, 2000; Webster, 2001). Moreover the practice of feeding relatively wet grass silage seems to add to the problems (Offer, Fisher, Kempson, and Logue, 2001; Offer, Leach, Brocklehurst and Logue, 2003). Also, with increasing herd size and yield there tends to be more housing, mixing of the cows into groups and so more opportunity for increased mechanical stresses on the claw (Leonard, O'Connell and O'Farrell, 1994, 1995; Logue *et al.*, 1999). Unfortunately even at grazing the farmer has the problem of gathering his ever-larger herd and moving it to his milking parlour. Not surprisingly the quality of the tracks has also been related to lameness (Harris, Hibburt, Anderson, Younis, Fitzpatrick, Dunn, Parsons and McBeath, 1988; Chesterton, Pfeiffer, Morris and Tanner, 1989; Leonard, Crilly and O'Farrell, 1998). It is suggested that tracks should be carefully maintained and reviewed annually before turnout.

Foot trimming and foot bathing have been long advocated as a means for limiting the problems of lameness (Arkins, 1981; Toussaint Raven, Haalstra and Peterse, 1985; Manson and Leaver, 1988; Manske, Hultgren and Bergsten, 2002). All the evidence from the literature is that they work (see Table 4) but there is relatively little reliable data concerning the relative merits of different foot bathing agents or the best frequency. Finally it is hardly surprising that buying in animals has

Table 4. Some environmental and nutritional risk factors for lameness* (of all types) and their estimated "strength" based on papers from the systematic review *http://www.cattle-lameness.com*

Environmental management factors increasing lameness in herds	*Strength evidence* %	*Cow management factors influencing lameness**	*Strength evidence* %
Poorly maintained tracks	73%	Poor/wet grass silage	100%
Reducing lying time through poor comfort	72%	Less lameness including hay in diet	80%
Hardness &/or abrasive of housing floor surface (e.g. cubicle vs. straw yd)	68%	High concentrate:forage ratio	75%
Increased wet and dirt on floor surface	64%	Less lameness with good stockmanship	72%
Increased buying-in replacements (closed)	63%	Less lameness with foot bathing	66%
Reduced exercise	63%	Less lameness with routine foot trimming	47%
Increased proportion of slatted floors	58%	Bigger herds (or groups)	47%
Increased average yield of herd	37%	Higher concentrate inputs	45%
Poor collection and management at milking	33%	Less with vitamin/minerals supplement	41%

*More lameness with risk factor unless stated

been found associated with an increase in infectious conditions such as digital dermatitis (Argaez-Rodriguez, Hird, Hernandez, Read and Rodriguez, 1997; Rodriguez-Lainz *et al.*, 1999; Wells, Garber and Wagner, 1999). Farmers again need to think more seriously about their biosecurity.

Some practical approaches to controlling lameness are summarised in Table 5. In this table we have attempted to aid the farmer by putting an estimated cost against the action. It is intended that they should start with the easiest and cheapest for their farm.

Conclusion

In conclusion the wellbeing and longevity of the cow is strongly influenced by three conditions, infertility, mastitis and lameness. It is hoped that this paper has highlighted a number of practical management strategies that will increase functional longevity and improve genetic selection for this parameter. In our opinion they will improve welfare and therefore safeguard the status of farm assurance within the UK. In the long-term this will protect our home market.

Acknowledgements

The authors gratefully acknowledge all their colleagues who have discussed this subject at length and especially Mark Hirst, Andrea Le Fevre, Nigel French, Sarah Brocklehurst, George Gettinby, Richard Laven and Alison Gibbs for their part in the systematic review of lameness and Andrea Le Fevre for access to Figure 6, They are also grateful to the various funding bodies who have provided financial support for the various studies referred to here. These include; the EU, the three Milk Marketing Boards in Scotland, ABN, the Animal Health Trust, MAFF, the Wellcome Trust, Milk Development Council, the Nuffield Foundation, BBSRC and, of course, the Scottish Office Agriculture, Environment and Fisheries Department.

References

Alban, L., Lawson, L.G. and Agger, J.F. (1995) Foul in the foot (interdigital necrobacillosis) in Danish dairy cows - frequency and possible risk factors. *Preventive Veterinary Medicine* 24, 73-82.

Anon. (1997) *Report on the Welfare of the Dairy Cow*. Farm Animal Welfare Council, MAFF Publication, Tolworth, UK, 1-95.

Anon (2002) *Preparing an Animal Health and Welfare Strategy for*

Table 5. Some on-farm strategies for limiting lameness in dairy cattle

Strategy	*Action*	*Comments*	*Likely cost*
Reduce infection	Immediate treatment of all conditions	Record types of lameness and all treatments	Low
	Specific targeted treatment footbath		Low
Ensure good claw shape/ condition	Regular foot trim	Trained personnel	Low
	Regular routine preventive foot bath	(wash feet first!)	Low
Animal factors	Season of calving	Input type/milk price	Medium
	Training to system	Culling policy heifers trained to cubicles etc.,	Medium Low
Reduce environmental impact	Lying comfort	Adequate bedding!	Low
	Good slurry system	Good comfortable cubicle design &/or adequate space per cow (including feed & water)	Expensive
Nutrition	Marry inputs to outputs to limit weight loss in early lactation	Limit weight loss post-calving esp., in heifers.	Low
	Seek highly palatable forages	Use mixed forages and aim for high DM	Low
	Avoid macro or micro-element deficiencies	Limit concentrate meals and align with forage	Low

Great Britain. A consultation document by UK Government, the Scottish Executive and the National Assmbly for Wales. DEFRA, UK, 1-19.

Argaez-Rodriguez, F. de J., Hird, D.W., Hernandez, J. de A., Read, D.H. and Rodriguez-Lainz, A. (1997) Papillomatous digital dermatitis on a commercial dairy farm in Mexicali, Mexico: incidence and effect on reproduction and milk production. *Preventive Veterinary Medicine* 32, 275-286.

Arkins, S. (1981) Lameness in dairy cows. *Irish Veterinary Journal* 35, 135-141 & 163-170.

Bergsten, C. and Herlin, A.H. (1995) Sole haemorrhages and heel horn erosion in dairy cows: the influence of housing system on their prevalence and severity. *Acta Veterinaria Scandinavica* 37, 395-408.

Boyd, H. and Reed, H.C.B. (1961a) Investigations into the incidence and causes of infertility in dairy cattle-fertility variations. *British Veterinary Journal* 117, 18-35.

Boyd, H. and Reed, H.C.B. (1961b) Investigations into the incidence and causes of infertility in dairy cattle-influence of some management factors affecting the semen and insemination conditions. *British Veterinary Journal* 117, 74-86.

Butler W. R. (2001) Nutritional effects on resumption of ovarian cyclicity and conception rate in postpartum dairy cows. In: *Fertility in the High Producing Dairy Cow.* Occasional Publication No. 26 (Volume 1), Edited by Diskin, M.G., British Society of Animal Science, pp. 133-145.

Chesterton, R.N., Pfeiffer, D.U., Morris, R.S., Tanner, C.M. (1989) Environmental and behavioural factors affecting the prevalence of foot lameness in New Zealand dairy herds - a case-control study. *New Zealand Veterinary Journal* 37, 135-142.

Clarkson, M.J., Downham, D.Y., Faull, W.B., Hughes, J.W., Manson, F.J., Merrit, J.B., Murray, R.D., Russell, W.B., Sutherst, J. and Ward, W.R. (1996) Incidence and prevalence of lameness in dairy cattle. *Veterinary Record* 138, 563-567.

Collick, D.W., Ward, W.R. and Dobson, H. (1989) Association between types of lameness and fertility. *Veterinary Record* 125, 103-106.

Cromie, A.R., Gordon, F.J., Kelleher, D.L. and Rath, M. (1998) Harnessing genetics for better profit. In: *Proceedings of the Northern Ireland Dairy conference,* Antrim, UK, Edited by Gordon F. and McIroy G., pp. 49-59.

Eshraghi, H.R., Zeitlin, I.J., Fitzpatrick, J., Ternent, T.H. and Logue, D.N. (1999) The release of Bradykinin in bovine mastitis. *Life Sciences* 64, 1675-1687.

Esslemont, R.J. and Kossaibati, M.A. (1997) Culling in 50 dairy herds in England. *Veterinary Record* 140, 36-39.

Faye, B. and Lescourret, F. (1989) Environmental factors associated with lameness in dairy cattle. *Preventive Veterinary Medicine* 7,

267-287.

Fitzpatrick, J. L., Young, F. J., Eckersall, D., Logue, D.N., Knight, C.J. and Nolan, A. (1998) Recognising and controlling pain and inflammation in mastitis. *British Mastitis Conference 1998,* pp. 36- 44.

Forbes, D., Gayton, S. and McGeogh, B. (1999) Improving the longevity of cows in the UK dairy herd. *Milk Development Council Longevity Report 97/R1/12, Final Report August 1999,* pp. 1-24.

Gunn, G. Stott, A.W., Humphry, R. Jones, G. (2000) Estimating the economic losses associated with BVD infection in the UK dairy herd. *Final Report, Milk Development Council Project No: 99/ R4/01.*

Harris, D.J., Hibburt, C.D., Anderson, G.A., Younis, P.J., Fitzpatrick, D.H., Dunn, A.C., Parsons, I W. and McBeath, N.R. (1988) The incidence, cost and factors associated with foot lameness in dairy-cattle in south-western Victoria. *Australian Veterinary Journal* **65**, 171-176.

Harvey, D. (2001) Whither Agriculture? *Farm Management* **10**, 751-772.

Hernandez, J., Shearer, J.K. and Webb, D.W. (2001) Effect of lameness on the calving-to-conception interval in dairy cows. *Journal of the American Veterinary Medical Association* **218**, 1611-1614.

Hirst, W.M. Le Fevre, A.M., Logue, D.N., Offer, J.E. Chaplin, S.J., Murray, R.D., Ward, W.R., French, N.P. (2002) Systematic Review of Lameness in Cattle. *The Veterinary Journal* **164**, 7-19.

Huang, Y.C., Shanks, R.D. and McCoy, G.C. (1995) Evaluation of fixed factors affecting hoof health. *Livestock Production Science* 44, 115-124

Knight, C., Beever, D.E. and Sorensen, A. (1999) Metabolic loads to be expected from different genotypes under different systems. In: *Metabolic Stress in the Dairy Cow.* Occasional Publication No. 24, Edited by Oldham, J.D., Simm, G., Green, A.F., Neilsen, B.L., Pryce, J.E. and Lawrence, T.L.J, British Society of Animal Science, pp. 27-35.

Knight, C.H., Fitzpatrick, J.L., Logue, D.N., Platt, D.J. Robertson, S. and Ternent, H.E. (2000) Efficacy of two non-antibiotic therapies oxytocin and topical liniment against experimentally-induced Staphylococcus aureus mastitis. *Veterinary Record* **146**, 311-316.

Kossaibati, M.A. and Esslemont, R.J. (1997) The costs of production disease in dairy herds in England. *The Veterinary Journal* 154, 41-51.

Larsen, H.D., Sloth, K.H., Elsberg, C., Enevoldsen, C., Pedersen, L.H., Eriksen, N.H.R., Aarestrup, F.M. and Jensen, N.E. (2000) The dynamics of Staphylococcus aureus intramammary infection in nine Danish dairy herds. *Veterinary Microbiology* 71, 89-101.

Le Fevre, A.M. (2003) Modelling and understanding claw horn lesions of dairy cattle. PhD Thesis, University of Strathclyde, UK.

Le Fevre, A.M., Hirst, W.M., French, N.P., Offer, J.E., Brocklehurst S., Gibbs A., Laven R., Gettinby, G. and Logue D.N. (2002) Using a systematic review of lameness in dairy cattle to develop an intervention study. In: *Proceedings of the Society of Veterinary Epidemiology and Preventive Medicine,* pp. 167-177.

Leonard, F.C., Crilly, J. and O'Farrell, K.J. (1998) Analysis of roadway surfaces on dairy farms and the relationship with lameness. In: *10th Symposium on Lameness in Dairy Cattle.* Edited by Lischer, Ch.J. and Ossent, P., pp 73-75.

Leonard, F.C., O'Connell, J. and O'Farrell, K. (1995) Effect of overcrowding on claw health in first-calved Friesian heifers. *British Veterinary Journal* **152**, 459-472.

Leonard, F.C., O'Connell, J. and O'Farrell, K. (1994) Effect of different housing conditions on behaviour and foot lesions in Friesian heifers. *Veterinary Record* **134**, 490-494.

Lindhe, B. and Philipson, J. (2001) The Scandinavian experience of including reproductive traits in breeding programmes. In: *Fertility in the High Producing Dairy Cow.* Occasional Publication No. 26 (Volume 1), Edited by Diskin, M.G., British Society of Animal Science, pp 251-261.

Livesey, C.T., Harrington, T., Johnston, A.M., May, S.A. and Metcalf, J.A. (1998) The effect of diet and housing on the development of sole haemorrhages, white line haemorrhages and heel erosions in Holstein heifers. *Animal Science* **67**, 9-16.

Livesey, C.T. and Fleming, F.L. (1984) Nutritional influences on laminitis, sole ulcer and bruised sole in Friesian cows. *Veterinary Record* **114**, 510-512.

Logue, D.N. (2002) A preliminary review of the effects of environment and behaviour on lameness in the dairy cow. In: *12th International Symposium on Lameness in Ruminants.* Edited by Shearer, J.K., pp. 18-26.

Logue, D.N. and Isbister, J. (1992) Bull infertility. In: *Bovine Medicine.* Edited by Andrews, A.H., Blackwell Scientific Publications, Oxford, UK, pp. 482-507.

Logue, D.N., Berry, R.J., Offer, J.E., Chaplin, S.J., Crawshaw, W.M., Leach, K.A., Ball, P.J.H. and Bax, J. (1999) Consequences of "metabolic load" for lameness and disease. In: *Metabolic Stress in the Dairy Cow.* Occasional Publication No. 24, Edited by Oldham, J.D., Simm, G., Green, A.F., Neilsen, B.L., Pryce, J.E. and Lawrence, T.L.J, British Society of Animal Science, pp 83-98.

Lucey, M.C. and Crooker, B.A. (2001) Physiological and genetic differences between low and high index dairy cows. In: *Fertility in the High Producing Dairy Cow.* Occasional Publication No. 26 (Volume 1), Edited by Diskin, M.G., British Society of Animal Science, pp223-236.

Manske, T., Hultgren, J. and Bergsten, C. (2002) The effect of claw trimming on the hoof health of Swedish dairy cattle. *Preventive*

Veterinary Medicine 54, 113-129.
Manson, F.J. and Leaver, J.D. (1988) The influence of dietary protein intake and of hoof trimming on lameness in dairy cattle. *Animal Production* 47, 191-199
O'Farrell, K.J. (1998) Changes in dairy cow fertility. *Cattle Practice* 6, 387-392.
O'Callaghan, D., Lozano, J.M., Fahey, J., Gath, V., Snijders, S. and Boland, M.P. 2001. In: *Fertility in the High Producing Dairy Cow.* Occasional Publication No. 26 (Volume 1), Edited by Diskin, M.G., British Society of Animal Science, pp.147-159.
Offer, J.E., McNulty, D. and Logue, D.N. (1999) Observations of lameness hoof conformation and development of lesions in dairy cattle over four lactations. *Veterinary Record* 147, 105-109.
Offer, J.E., Fisher, G.E.J., Kempson, S.E. and Logue, D.N. (2001) The effect of feeding grass silage in early pregnancy on claw health during first lactation. *The Veterinary Journal* 161, 186-193.
Offer, J.E. Leach, K.A., Brocklehurst, S. and Logue, D.N. (2003) Effect of type of forage fed to dairy young stock on claw horn lesion development during rearing and first lactation. *The Veterinary Journal* 165, 221-227
Peterse, D.J., Korver, S., Oldenbroek, J.K. and Talmon, F. P. (1984) Relationship between levels of concentrate feeding and the incidence of sole ulcers in dairy cattle. *Veterinary Record* 115, 629-630.
Pryce, J.E., Veerkamp, R.F., Thompson, R., Hill, W.G. and Simm, G. (1998) Genetic parameters of common health disorders and measures of fertility in Holstein Friesian dairy cattle. *Animal Science* 65, 353-360.
Rodriguez-Lainz, A. Melendez-Retamal, P., Hird, D.W., Read, D.H. and Walker, R.L. (1999) Farm- and host-level risk factors for digital dermatitis in Chilean dairy cattle. *Preventive Veterinary Medicine* 42, 87-97.
Rodriguez-Lainz, A.J., Hird, D.W., Carpenter, T.E. and Read, D.H. (1996) Case control study of papillomatous digital dermatitis in Southern California dairy farms. *Preventive Veterinary Medicine* 28, 117-131.
Royal, M.D., Darwash, A.O., Flint, A.P.F., Webb, R., Williams, J.A. and Lamming, G.E. (2000) Declining fertility in dairy cattle: changes in traditional and endocrine parameters of fertility. *Animal Science* 70, 487-501.
Ryan, D.P. and Mee, J.F. (1994) Irish dairy herd fertility research *Cattle Practice* 2, 241-249.
Schaik, van G., Dijkhuizen, A.A., Benedictus, G., Barkema, H.W. and Koole J.L. (1998) Exploratory study on the economic value of a closed farming system on Dutch farms. *Veterinary Record* 142, 240-242.
Sinclair, M.C., Nielsen, B.L. Oldham, J.D. and Reid, H.W. (1999)

Consequences for immune functions of metabolic adaptations to load. In: *Metabolic Stress in the Dairy Cow.* Occasional Publication No. 24, Edited by Oldham, J.D., Simm, G., Green, A.F., Neilsen, B.L., Pryce, J.E. and Lawrence, T.L.J, British Society of Animal Science, pp. 113-118.

Sreenan, J.M., Diskin, M.G. and Morris, D.G. (2001) Embryo survival rate in cattle: a major limitation to the achievement of high fertility. In: *Fertility in the High Producing Dairy Cow.* Occasional Publication No. 26 (Volume 1), Edited by Diskin, M.G., British Society of Animal Science, pp 93-104.

Stott, A.W. (1994) The economic advantage of longevity in the dairy cow. *Journal of Agricultural Economics* 45, 113-122.

Stott, A.W., Veerkamp, R.F. and Wassell, T.R. (1999) The economics of fertility in the dairy herd. *Animal Science* 68, 49-57.

Stott, A.W., Gunn, G.J., Humphry, R.W., Chase-Topping, M., Jones, G., Berry, R.J., Richardson, H. and Logue D.N. (2000) What to do with Staph cows? Guidelines for the control of *S. aureus* subclinical mastitis by culling using recommendations based on a bio-economic computer model. In: *British Mastitis Conference.* Institute for Animal Health and Milk Development Council, UK, pp. 44-55.

Stott, A.W., Jones, G.M., Gunn, G.J., Chase-Topping, M., Humphry, R.W., Richardson, H. and Logue, D.N. (2002) Optimum replacement policies for control of subclinical mastitis due to *S. aureus* in dairy cows. *Journal of Agricultural Economics* 53, 627-644.

Thatcher, W.W., Binelli, M., Arnold, D., Mattos, R., Badinga, L., Moreira,F., Staples, C.R. and Guzeloglu, A. (2001) Endocrine and physiological events from ovulation to establishment of pregnancy in cattle. In: *Fertility in the High Producing Dairy Cow.* Occasional Publication No. 26 (Volume 1), Edited by Diskin, M.G., British Society of Animal Science, pp 81-91.

Toussaint Raven, E., Haalstra, R.T. and Peterse, D.J. (1985) Cattle Footcare and claw trimming. (English translation of Dutch originally published 1977) *Farming Press Ipswich 1985*, pp. 1-126.

Veerkamp, R.F., Hill, W.G., Stott, A.W., Brotherstone S., and Simm, G. (1994) Selection for longevity and yield in dairy cows using transmitting abilities for type and yield. *Animal Science* 61, 189-197.

Watson, E.D., Jones, P.C. and Saunders, R.W. (1987) Effect of factors associated with insemination on calving rate in dairy cows. *Veterinary Record* 121, 256-258.

Webb, R. Garnsworthy, P.C., Gong, J.G., Robinson, R.S. and Wathes. D.C. (1999) Consequences for reproductive function of metabolic adaptation to load. In: *Metabolic Stress in the Dairy Cow.*

Occasional Publication No. 24, Edited by Oldham, J.D., Simm, G., Green, A.F., Neilsen, B.L., Pryce, J.E. and Lawrence, T.L.J, British Society of Animal Science, pp. 92-122.

Webb, R., Garnsworthy, P., Gong, J.G., Gutterrez, C.G., Logue, D.N., Crawshaw, W.M. and Robinson, J.J. (1997) Nutritional influence on subfertility in cattle. *Cattle Practice* 5, 361-367.

Webster A.J.F. (2001) The effect of housing and two forage diets on the development of claw horn lesions in dairy cows at first calving and in first lactation. *The Veterinary Journal* 162, 56-65.

Webster, A.J.F. (1995) Welfare strategies in future selection and management strategies. In: *Breeding and Feeding the High Genetic Merit Dairy Cow.* Occasional publication No 19, Edited by Lawrence, T.J.L., Gordon, F.J. and Carson, A, British Society of Animal Science, pp. 87- 93.

Wells, S.J., Trent, A.M., Marsh, W.E. and Robinson, R.A. (1993) Prevalence and severity of lameness in lactating dairy cattle in a sample of Minnesota and Wisconsin herds. *Journal of the American Veterinary Medical Association* 202, 78-82.

Wells, S.J., Garber, L.P. and Wagner, B.A. (1999) Papillamatous digital dermatitis and associated risk factors in US dairy herds. *Preventive Veterinary Medicine* 38, 11-24.

Whay, H.R., Main, D.C.J. Green, L.E. and Webster, A.J.F. (2002) In: *12th International Symposium on Lameness in Ruminants.* Edited by Shearer, J.K., pp. 355-358.

Whitaker, D., Kelly, J.M., and Smith, S. (2000) Disposal rates and disease rates in 340 British dairy herds. *Veterinary Record* 146, 363-367.

Yalcin, C., Stott, A.W., Logue, D.N. and Gunn, G.J. (1999) The economic impact of mastitis-control procedures used in Scottish dairy herds with high bulk-tank somatic-cell counts. *Preventive Veterinary Medicine* 41, 135-149.

Young, G.B., Waddington, D., Sales, D.I., Bradley, J.S. and Spooner, R.L. (1983) Culling and wastage in dairy cows in East Anglia. *Veterinary Record* 113, 107-111.

5

OPTIMISING MILK COMPOSITION

Adam L. Lock*‡ and Kevin J. Shingfield†
*Division of Agricultural Sciences, University of Nottingham, Loughborough, LE12 5RD. † Centre for Dairy Research, Department of Animal Science, University of Reading, Earley Gate, Reading, RG6 6AR, U.K

Introduction

During recent decades, the UK dairy industry has had to adjust to the introduction of milk quotas in 1984, the deregulation of milk markets in 1994, and accommodate changes in the demand for dairy products. The combination of these factors, in addition to Bovine Spongiform Encephalopathy and Foot and Mouth disease, and a fall in milk price has inevitably resulted in a restructuring of the industry, but also reinforced the need for all sectors of the industry to respond to the prevailing economic climate and changes in consumer preferences. Producing milk with a composition that is consistent with the demand for milk constituents, not only improves biological efficiency, but also increases the profitability of the dairy industry (Kennelly, 1996). The success of attempts to match supply with demand is ultimately dependent on the manipulation of milk composition in line with market forces. Improvements in animal genetics can be used to align production with demand in the long term, but does not offer a short to medium term solution. In contrast, nutrition can be used to alter milk composition and facilitate rapid responses to changes in milk markets, but the potential benefits are dependent on the development of nutritional strategies leading to the production of milk with a composition consistent with requirements.

Following the introduction of quotas within the European Union in 1984, there has been considerable interest in altering the fat to protein ratio of milk. Once the national butterfat base level has been exceeded, a decrease of 0.1 g/kg in milk fat content would permit 0.0018 proportionate increases in milk volume. The ability to increase milk production within the constraints of imposed quotas and changes in milk-pricing schemes has become increasingly important. Nutritional factors affecting the secretion of milk constituents are well established

‡Current address: Department of Animal Science, Cornell University, 262 Morrison Hall, Ithaca, NY 14853, USA

(DePeters and Cant, 1992, Storry, 1981, Sutton, 1989, Thomas and Chamberlain, 1984), whilst more recent research has provided a further insight into the effect of diet on milk composition, taking into account the increased use of alternative forages and protein crops for milk production. These findings, in addition to the role of nutrition on the regulation of milk fat synthesis, manipulation of milk fatty acid composition and enriching functional components in milk are currently reviewed in the context of developing nutritional strategies for optimising milk composition.

Changes in demand for milk and dairy products

During the last fifty years consumption of liquid milk and dairy products has dramatically changed. In the early post-war years production was barely capable of satisfying demand for liquid milk and the manufacture of dairy products was often dependent on imported materials (Thomas and Chamberlain, 1984). Markets recognised this demand and producers were encouraged to maximise milk fat production. However, the demand for milk fat has declined in recent years with the result that producers receive a higher premium for protein than fat. Demand for milk fat has decreased due to reduced butter consumption (Table 1) arising from increased prevalence of alternative vegetable spreads and margarines, and consumer preference for skimmed and semi-skimmed milk (Table 1).

Reduced demand for whole fat milk can be considered as a reflection of greater consumer awareness of an association between dietary fat intake and the risk of coronary heart disease following the publication of the Committee on Medical Aspects of Food Policy (COMA) reports in 1984 and 1994. The fall in demand for milk fat in liquid milk has, to some extent, been compensated for, by an increase in the consumption of cheese (Table 1), but butter sales have failed to recover.

Synthesis of milk constituents

Milk fat, protein and lactose are synthesised in the mammary gland from precursors absorbed from the peripheral circulation. From the onset of lactation, synthesis of milk constituents occurs at such high rates that without strict regulation metabolic problems would rapidly be encountered (Bequette, Backwell and Crompton, 1998). Establishment and co-ordination of these processes through acute and chronic interactions between nutrients, hormones and tissues permit high rates of milk production while still allowing nutrients to be partitioned to tissues other than the mammary gland. Such adaptations have the overall effect of providing the appropriate quantity and balance of

Table 1. Consumption of milk and dairy products in the United Kingdom (g/person/week, unless otherwise stated [1]).

	1960	1965	1970	1975	1980	1985	1990	1995	2000
Liquid wholemilk (ml)	2750	2756	2631	2709	2364	1888	1232	812	664
Skimmed milk[2]				7	20	244	709	1103	1138
Total milk and cream	2921	2949	2887	2913	2604	2348	2169	2170	2081
Yoghurt and fromage frais				24	48	74	97	127	141
Total cheese	86	91	102	107	110	111	113	108	110
Butter	161	173	170	160	115	80	46	36	39

[1] From Department for Environment Food and Rural Affairs available at: www.defra.gov.uk/esg/m_natstats.htm
[2] Skimmed milk includes dairy desserts and other milk until 1983

nutrients for milk synthesis (Bauman, 2000). Metabolic pathways for the synthesis of fat, protein and lactose in the mammary gland are presented in Figure 1.

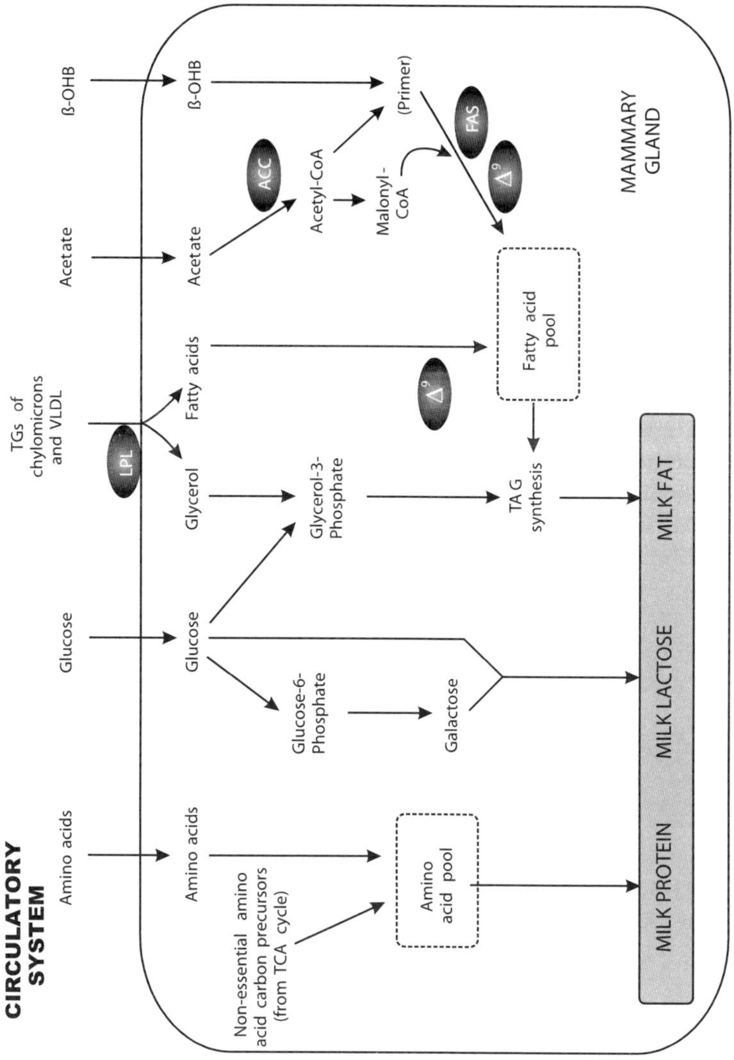

Figure 1. Milk synthesis in the mammary gland. Appreviations used. β-OHB: β-hydroxybutyrate; LPL: lipoprotein lipase; ACC: acetyl-CoA carboxylase; FAS: fatty acid synthetase and Δ^9: Δ^9-desaturase.

Milk fat

Milk fat contains a complex mixture of lipids, primarily in the form of triacylglycerides (proportionately 0.98), with the remainder as di- and monoacylglycerides, phopholipids, cholesterol, and non-esterified fatty acids (NEFA) (Christie, 1995). Fatty acids (FA) secreted in milk are derived directly from the peripheral circulation and *de novo* synthesis in the mammary gland. Direct uptake typically contributes to about 60 % of total mammary FA secretion (Chilliard, Ferlay, Mansbridge and Doreau, 2000). *De novo* synthesis accounts for all $C_{4:0}$ to $C_{12:0}$, most of the $C_{14:0}$ and about half of $C_{16:0}$ secreted in milk, while all C_{18} and longer chained FA are derived entirely from circulating blood lipids (Hawke and Taylor, 1995). In contrast to milk, other ruminant lipids do not contain appreciable amounts of short and medium chain FA (Moore and Christie, 1981).

Figure 1 provides an overview of the metabolic pathways for FA synthesis in the mammary gland. *De novo* synthesis has an absolute requirement for carbon in the form of acetyl-CoA, two key enzymes (acetyl-CoA carboxylase and fatty acid synthetase) and a supply of NADPH reducing equivalents (Hawke and Taylor, 1995). Acetate, and to a lesser extent ß-hydroxybutyrate, contribute to the initial four carbons units required for FA synthesis. Acetate is converted to acetyl Co A in the cytosol and incorporated into FA via the malonyl-Co A pathway, whereas ß-hydroxybutyrate is incorporated directly following activation to butyl Co A (Murphy, 2000). Conversion of acetate to acetyl-CoA via acetyl-CoA carboxylase is considered to be the rate-limiting step (Bauman and Davis, 1974).

Fatty acid synthetase consists of a large enzyme complex and is responsible for chain elongation. Acetyl, butyl and malonyl-Co A condense within the fatty acid synthetase complex and chain elongation occurs through continual loading of additional malonyl-Co A groups. A distinctive feature of the bovine mammary gland is the ability to release FA from the synthetase complex at various stages, resulting in the secretion of a wide range of short and medium chain FA in milk.

The mammary gland is also capable of utilising preformed FAs through the uptake of plasma NEFA and triacylglyceride rich lipoproteins (Chilliard *et al.*, 2000). Triacylglycerides associated with plasma chylomicrons and very low-density lipoproteins (VLDL) in particular, are the major transport mechanisms responsible for supplying FA to the mammary gland. Mammary uptake of low-density lipoproteins (LDL) and high-density lipoproteins (HDL) is relatively limited (Offer, Speake, Dixon and Marsden, 2001a) and accounts for the low transfer of absorbed long-chain FA into milk (Chilliard, Ferlay and Doreau, 2001). Due to extensive metabolism of dietary unsaturated FA in the rumen, $C_{18:0}$ is the predominant long chain FA available for incorporation into milk fat. However, *cis*-9 $C_{18:1}$ secretion exceeds $C_{18:0}$ uptake due to the activity of stearoyl Co A (Δ-9) desaturase activity in mammary secretory cells (Kinsella, 1972). Introduction of a *cis*-9 double bond is thought to occur in order to ensure the fluidity of milk for efficient secretion from the mammary gland (Grummer, 1991). Conversion of $C_{18:0}$ to *cis*-9 $C_{18:1}$ is the predominant precursor:product of the Δ-9 desaturase, transforming proportionately 0.40 of $C_{18:0}$ taken up by the mammary gland (Chilliard *et al.*, 2000). Activity is not confined to $C_{18:0}$, such that $C_{14:0}$ and $C_{16:0}$ are also desaturated, the latter accounting for proportionately 0.20 of $C_{18:0}$ conversion. Further studies have shown that both *trans*-11 $C_{18:1}$ (Griinari, Corl, Lacy, Chouinard, Nurmela and Bauman, 2000) and *trans*-7 $C_{18:1}$ (Corl, Baumgard, Griinari, Delmonte, Morehouse, Yuraweczc and Bauman 2002, Piperova, Sampugna, Teter, Kalscheur, Yurawecz, Ku, Morehouse and Erdman, 2002) are also converted resulting in the formation of *cis*-9, *trans*-11 $C_{18:2}$ and *trans*-7, *cis*-9 $C_{18:2}$, respectively.

Incorporation of preformed and FA synthesised *de novo* into triacylglycerides occurs via the glycerol-3-phosphate pathway (Hawke and Taylor, 1995). Between 50 and 60% of glycerol-3-phosphate is estimated to come from glucose, with the remainder from glycerol liberated during lipolysis of plasma triacylglycerides (Bauman and Davis, 1974). In spite of sequential addition to the glycerol backbone, FAs are not randomly distributed within triacylglycerides. Saturated FA are predominately located in the sn-1 position, shorter chained and unsaturated FA at sn-2, while C_{18} and long chained FA are located in the sn-3 position (Demeyer and Doreau, 1999).

Milk protein

Milk protein constitutes about 95 % of total milk nitrogen, and contains caseins (α, ß, κ and γ), whey proteins (ß-lactoglobulin and α-lactalbumin), serum albumin and immunoglobulins. Casein accounts for between 76 and 86% of total milk protein (DePeters and Cant, 1992), while the ratio of casein to total protein is largely independent of nutrition and stage of lactation (Coulon, Hurtaud, Remond and Vérité, 1998). Non-protein nitrogen fractions (urea, peptides, amino acids, creatinine and purine metabolites) appear in milk as a result of diffusion from the peripheral circulation, while milk proteins other than serum albumin and immunoglobulins are synthesised in mammary epithelial cells from amino acid (AA) precursors.

Even though total AA uptake can account for milk protein secretion (Mepham, 1976), extraction from arterial blood and output in milk is not balanced for all AA. Uptake of several non-essential AA (methionine, histidine, phenylalanine and tryptophan) is lower than output (Clark, 1975, DePeters and Cant, 1992, Bequette, Backwell and Crompton, 1998), whilst the secretion of others (most notably branched chain AA and arginine) is considerably lower than extraction due to extensive oxidation in the mammary gland (Mepham, 1982). Utilisation of AA by the mammary gland occurs following uptake from the peripheral circulation by secretory cells and subsequent intracellular protein synthesis within the endoplasmic reticulum (Mepham, 1987). Synthesis of milk proteins has an absolute requirement for ATP produced during the oxidation of acetate, certain AA and glucose (Erasmus, Hermansen and Rulquin, 2001).

Positive linear relationships between arterio-venous differences and arterial essential AA concentrations have often been reported (e.g. Hanigan, Calvert, DePeters, Reis and Baldwin, 1992, Metcalf, Beever, Sutton, Wray-Cohen, Evans, Humphries, Blackwell, Bequette and MacRae, 1994) indicating that uptake is largely dependent on circulating concentrations. However, plasma concentrations are not the sole determinant of uptake, since mammary blood flow and AA requirements for milk protein synthesis also have an influence, thus enabling the mammary gland to respond to changes in essential AA supply (Cant, Berthiaume, Lapierre, Luimes, McBride and Pacheco, 2002, Mackle Dwyer, Ingvartsen, Chouinard, Ross and Bauman, 2000). Whilst the mammary gland is capable of altering extraction rates, the extent of compensation is finite and therefore, under certain situations, milk protein synthesis can be limited by AA supply. In addition to AA supply, there is increasing evidence that milk protein synthesis can be modified in response to alterations in endocrine controls, principally insulin and insulin-like growth factor (Mackle and Bauman, 1998).

Milk lactose

Lactose is the main osmotic constituent of milk and is responsible for regulation of water secretion and therefore milk volume. Much less attention has been paid to manipulation of lactose concentrations compared with milk fat and protein, because nutrition has limited and generally inconsistent effects (Sutton, 1989), and this constituent is not recognised within milk-pricing schemes. However, lactose is important in terms of nutrient economy because a high proportion (0.85) is derived from plasma glucose (Bickerstaffe, Annison and Linzell, 1974). Even though the effect of nutrition is rather limited, milk lactose content has been shown to decrease in response to intra-ruminal infusions of butyrate (Huhtanen, Miettinen and Ylinen, 1993, Miettinen and Huhtanen, 1996) indicating that the mammary gland can, to some extent, regulate lactose synthesis.

Dietary manipulation of milk constituents

Owing to changes in the demand for milk constituents, protein is more valuable to producers and processors. Understandably there has been an interest in increasing the protein to fat ratio of milk. Greater changes can be effected through reductions in milk fat content than increases in milk protein concentrations. However, producers can be penalised for the production of milk with a fat content below a certain threshold, and therefore the ability to enhance milk protein content is also important. Milk composition can be manipulated by nutritional means or through exploitation of naturally occurring genetic variation. Genetic improvement has historically been achieved utilising between- (cross-breeding) or within-(selection) breed variation, whilst recent advances in genetic engineering offer the promise of changes not previously possible using traditional nutritional and genetic approaches (Karatzas and Turner, 1997, Wall, Kerr and Bondioli, 1997). The impact of nutrition and genetic improvements are often considered independently, but both have an impact on milk composition. Nutrition can be used effectively to manipulate milk fat content, but concentrations of milk protein are much less responsive (Sutton, 1989). In general, genetic selection has a greater long-term impact on milk protein than nutrition.

Milk protein

Milk protein content is dependent on both breed and stage of lactation in addition to nutrition. Breeds that produce milk with a high fat content also have higher protein concentrations, but the ratio of protein to fat is lower for Channel Island breeds compared with the Ayrshire, Holstein or Friesian (Murphy and O'Mara, 1993). Immediately post-calving milk protein concentrations are extremely high and approach levels of 200 g/kg due to the secretion of immunoglobulins derived from the peripheral circulation. Concentrations decline rapidly during the first five days postpartum and continue to decrease at a much slower rate reaching the lowest levels between 35 and 70 days postpartum. Thereafter, milk protein content tends to increase with advances in lactation (DePeters and Cant, 1992). In addition to changes during lactation, parity also affects milk protein content. Concentrations of milk protein decrease in animals above three years of age, such that across five successive lactations a proportionate 0.04 reduction can be expected (Erasmus, Hermansen and Rulquin, 2001).

In contrast with milk fat, the impact of nutrition on milk protein content is poorly defined. In general, milk protein content tends to increase with increases in energy intake from carbohydrates (Coulon and Remond, 1991, Emery, 1978), but decrease when relatively high levels of lipids are included in the diet (DePeters and Cant, 1992, Sutton, 1989, Wu and Huber, 1994). Dietary protein supplements (Chamberlain, Martin and Robertson, 1989, Santos, Santos, Theurer and Huber, 1998, Thomas and Rae, 1988) consistently increase milk protein secretion but have variable effects on milk protein content. Similarly, milk protein responses to post-ruminal infusions of casein (Clark, 1975, Hanigan, Cant, Weakly and Beckett, 1998, Whitelaw, Milne, Ørskov and Smith, 1986), individual AA (Cant *et al., 2002,* Rulquin, Pisulewski, Vérité and Guinard, 1993), glucose or starch (Reynolds, Sutton and Beever, 1997, Thomas and Chamberlain, 1984) have also been unpredictable. A number of comprehensive reviews have considered the impact of nutrition and feeding management on milk protein synthesis (e.g. Chamberlain, Martin and Robertson, 1989, DePeters and Cant, 1992, Murphy and O'Mara, 1993, Thomas and Chamberlain, 1984). During the intervening years more data has become available to assess the potential of developing nutritional strategies for manipulating milk protein content.

Amino acid supply

Numerous studies have shown that arterial essential AA concentrations and milk protein synthesis increase in response to abomasal infusions of casein (e.g. Hanigan, Bequette, Crompton and France, 2001) leading to the general conclusion that the AA composition of protein entering the duodenum is the single most important nutritional factor influencing milk protein content (Erasmus, Hermansen and Rulquin, 2001). Positive linear relationships between arterio-venous differences and arterial concentrations (e.g. Hanigan *et al.*, 1992, Metcalf *et al.*, 1994) indicate that mammary uptake of essential AA is dependent on arterial concentrations. For a given mammary blood flow, mammary AA uptake and milk protein synthesis can be improved through increases in arterial AA concentration (DePeters and Cant, 1992, Miettinen and Huhtanen, 1997). Enhancing arterial AA concentrations underpin nutritional strategies for enhancing milk protein content by promoting increases in AA availability to the mammary gland and/or improving the supply of essential AA that limit milk protein synthesis.

In ruminant animals the quantity of AA available for absorption is determined by the quantity of microbes synthesised in the rumen, the amount of dietary protein escaping degradation in the rumen, and to a lesser extent by endogenous protein reaching the duodenum (Satter, 1986). On most diets, microbial protein is the major component of duodenal protein accounting for proportionately between 0.42 and 0.93 of the total protein flux entering the small intestine (Stern, 1986). While a number of factors including rumen outflow rate, microbial maintenance coefficient, feeding level, diet, defaunation, ionophores and branch chain FA influence the energetic efficiency of microbial protein synthesis (EMPS), the supply of AA derived from rumen microbes is essentially a function of digestible organic matter intake (Shingfield, 2000).

Development of nutritional strategies to increase AA supply by improved EMPS has received much less attention compared with dietary protein supplements (Beever, 1993). Much of this can be attributed to the difficulties of measuring microbial protein synthesis (Broderick and

Merchen, 1992, Shingfield, 2000), numerous factors that affect EMPS (Dewhurst, Davies and Merry, 2000) and the inadequacies of techniques used to determine the rate and extent of OM fermentation in the rumen (Dewhurst, Hepper and Webster, 1995). EMPS is lower for grass silage (mean 23 g microbial N/kg organic matter apparently digested in the rumen (AOMDR)) than for fresh grass (30-45) or maize silage (45) (Agricultural Research Council (ARC), 1984). More recent data indicates that while the value of grass silage is probably underestimated (mean 30), EMPS is generally higher for diets based on whole crop cereal (36) or maize silages (48) and lower for legume silages (20; Givens and Rulquin, 2002), Figure 2). For maize silage based diets EMPS appears to be independent of inclusion rate, suggesting that replacing grass silage with maize silage could be used as a nutritional strategy for increasing AA supply (Givens and Rulquin, 2002).

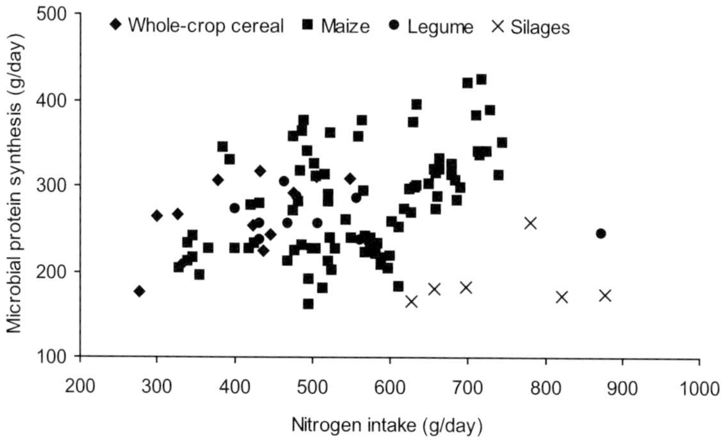

Figure 2. Relationship between nitrogen intake and microbial nitrogen supply. Adapted from Givens and Rulquin (2002).

Since protein in grass silage is extensively degraded in the rumen it has been argued that EMPS could be improved by a more synchronous release of energy and nitrogen in the rumen (Rooke, Lee and Armstrong, 1987, Siddons, Nolan, Beever and MacRae, 1985, Sinclair, Garnsworthy, Newbold and Buttery, 1993, Syrjälä, 1972). While this is an attractive hypothesis the evidence is to support this view is equivocal. For example, constant ruminal infusions of sucrose have been more effective in reducing ammonia nitrogen concentrations and stimulating microbial protein synthesis than twice daily supplements, that theoretically provide a more synchronous supply of energy and nitrogen in the rumen (Khalili and Huhtanen, 1991). In reviewing the available literature, Chamberlain and Choung (1995) concluded that there is no convincing evidence of the need for a close synchrony of energy and nitrogen release in the rumen for efficient microbial protein synthesis. It appears that formulating concentrate supplements to provide a constant supply of energy in the rumen appears to be the best strategy for optimising microbial protein supply on grass silage based diets (Henning, Steyen and Meissner, 1993).

Microbial AA composition has often (e.g. Martin, Bernard and Michalet-Doreau, 1996, Hanigan *et al.*, 1998, Volden and Harstad, 1998; Volden, Mydland and Harstad, 1999), but not in all cases (Clark, Klusmeyer and Cameron, 1992), been reported to be relatively constant. In spite of differences in AA content and contribution of individual microbial fractions, the AA profile of microbial protein entering the omasal canal is essentially independent of diet (Korhonen, Ahvenjärvi, Vanhatalo and Huhtanen, 2002). However, microbial protein alone is unable to satisfy the AA requirements of high-yielding dairy cows (Clark, 1975, Oldham, 1984, Ørskov and Reid, 1985) and therefore dietary protein supplements are used to improve the supply and/or balance of AA available for absorption (e.g. Jacobs and McAllan, 1992, Korhonen *et al.*, 2002, O' Mara, Murphy and Rath, 1998, Zerbini, Polan and Herbein, 1988).

Ingested protein entering the rumen is hydrolysed into peptides and amino acids by microbial proteases with the majority of AA being deaminated to ammonia, the extent of which is primarily governed by protein structure and rumen residence time (Beever, 1993). Understandably there has been considerable interest in replacing protein supplements of relatively high degradability with less degradable sources to increase the flow of AA entering the duodenum. Examination of data derived from a large number of studies has shown that replacement of soyabean meal with less degradable protein supplements does not necessarily guarantee an improvement in total protein or essential AA supply (Santos *et al.*, 1998), that can attributed to reduced microbial protein synthesis and/or poor digestibility or low essential AA content of protein escaping ruminal degradation. Similarly, supplements of rapeseed expeller or heat-treated rapeseed meal that have a lower degradability in the rumen compared with conventional rapeseed meal have not consistently increased milk protein output or concentration (Rinne, Jaakkola, Varvikko and Huhtanen, 1999a, Tuori, 1992).

Responses to protein supplements

Numerous studies have been conducted to examine the effects of both the amount and type of dietary protein on milk production (Chamberlain, Martin and Robertson, 1989, Thomas and Rae, 1988, Santos *et al.*, 1998). In general, dietary protein supplements increase milk protein output, as a result of higher milk yields rather than increases in milk protein content (Table 2). Responses are often variable and depend on both the source and level of supplementary protein, and also the composition of the basal ration. The importance of dietary protein source was recently demonstrated in a comparison of milk production responses to increases crude protein derived from grass silage, urea, wheat gluten meal or heat-treated rapeseed expeller (Shingfield, Jaakkola and Huhtanen, 2001). Higher applications of N fertilizer depressed milk protein content, urea supplements only increased milk protein output with low protein silage, while responses to wheat gluten meal were much lower for high compared with low protein silage. In contrast, responses to rapeseed expeller were independent of silage protein content. The level of protein in the diet is also an important determinant of milk protein responses, since incremental increases in protein intake (Figure 3) or infusions of casein in the abomasum (e.g. Whitelaw *et al.*, 1986) are partitioned towards milk protein synthesis with diminishing efficiency.

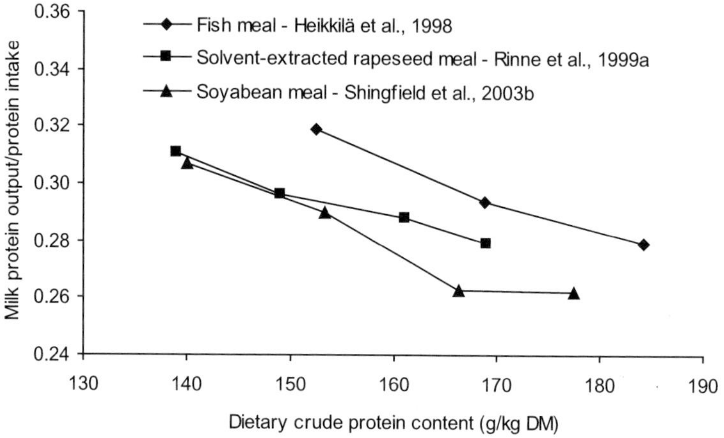

Figure 3. Association between dietary crude protein content and the partitioning of dietary protein towards milk protein synthesis in cows fed grass-silage based diets. Increases in protein content attained using various protein supplements.

In most cases dietary protein supplements stimulate higher forage DM intakes (Chamberlain, Martin and Robertson, 1989, Thomas and Rae, 1988) that have often been thought to account for the improvements in milk protein secretion (Sutton, 1989). Higher DM intakes also increase energy supply known to influence the milk protein content. For example, milk protein responses to post-ruminal casein infusions have almost doubled when energy intakes were increased from 85 to 100 % of predicted requirements (Rulquin, 1982). However, marginal increases in ME intake are often unable to explain the increase in milk energy secretion when protein supplements are included in the diet, suggesting that at least part of the milk protein response is also related to improvements in the balance of AA to energy at the tissue level.

Responses to amino acids

Since the profile of absorbed AA is considered to be the major factor influencing milk protein secretion, research has been directed towards determining the relative deficiencies of individual AA. Numerous studies involving abomasal AA infusions have implicated lysine and methionine as first and second limiting for milk and milk protein synthesis on most diets (e.g. Rulquin and Vérité, 1993, Schwab, Satter and Clay, 1976).

Table 2. Milk production responses to dietary protein supplements

Protein Source	Dietary CP content (g/kg DM)	Mean response per 100 g increase in dietary CP intake [a]				Reference
		Milk yield (g)	Protein content (g/kg)	Protein output (g/day)	Protein:fat ratio	
Fish meal	170-210	250	0.05	9.8	0.019	Bruckental *et al.*, 1989
Fish meal	129-186	412	0.04	14.8	-	Chamberlain *et al.*, 1989
Fish meal	165-200	362	0.35	15.0	0.009	Gordon and Small, 1990
Fish meal	129-152	444	0.23	20.1	0.009	Huhtanen *et al.*, 1993
Fish meal	152-184	145	0.18	10.5	0.003	Heikkilä *et al.*, 1998
Fish meal	167-189	450	0.12	16.5	0.008	Keady and Murphy, 1996
Fish meal	156-169	473	0.37	22.6	0.013	O'Mara *et al.*, 1998
Soyabean meal	151-189	308	0.15	15.6	-0.005	Kaim *et al.*, 1987
Soyabean meal	170-210	73	0.00	2.3	-0.004	Bruckental *et al.*, 1989
Soyabean meal	129-190	310	0.04	12.0	-	Chamberlain *et al.*, 1989
Soyabean meal	167-197	154	0.09	6.5	0.006	Peoples and Gordon, 1989
Soyabean meal	142-183	237	0.17	9.9	0.008	Cody *et al.*, 1990
Soyabean meal	161-181	218	0.12	11.2	0.001	Tuori, 1992
Soyabean meal	143-174	176	0.15	9.6	0.009	Metcalf *et al.*, 1994
Soyabean meal	157-170	400	0.29	17.6	0.012	O'Mara, Murphy and Rath, 1998
Soyabean meal	158-177	227	0.34	18.1	0.016	Kim *et al.*, 2001a
Soyabean meal	186-227	301	0.05	10.6	-0.002	Broderick *et al.*, 2002
Soyabean meal	140-177	274	0.04	11.3	0.003	Shingfield *et al.*, 2003b.
Protected soyabean meal	151-189	253	-0.28	5.5	-0.005	Kaim *et al.*, 1987
Protected soyabean meal	141-191	175	0.27	7.4	-	Metcalf *et al.*, 1996

Table 2. continued

Protein Source	*Dietary CP content (g/kg DM)*	*Mean response per 100 g increase in dietary CP intake* [a]				*Reference*
		Milk yield (g)	*Protein content (g/kg)*	*Protein output (g/day)*	*Protein:fat ratio*	
Rapeseed meal	161-182	405	0.02	14.7	0.000	Tuori, 1992
Rapeseed meal	142-160	629	-0.20	15.2	0.004	Bertilsson *et al.*, 1994
Rapeseed meal	127-149	369	0.07	13.9	0.003	Huhtanen, 1994
Rapeseed meal	139-169	444	0.05	16.3	0.002	Rinne *et al.*, 1999a
Rapeseed meal	144-165	385	-0.01	13.2	-0.002	Kokkonen *et al.*, 2000
Heat-treated rapeseed meal	141-160	182	0.14	9.6	0.008	Bertilsson *et al.*, 1994
Heat-treated rapeseed meal	127-150	392	0.10	14.9	0.005	Huhtanen, 1994
Heat-treated rapeseed expeller	139-164	556	0.00	17.2	0.001	Rinne *et al.*, 1999a
Heat-treated rapeseed expeller	140-177	452	-0.01	15.5	0.006	Shingfield *et al.*, 2001

[a] Responses calculated as the difference between treatment controls and protein supplemented diets and expressing the response per 100 g of additional protein intake. For studies where several protein supplementation levels were evaluated, responses were calculated as the mean across all treatments.

In cases where maize and maize by-products provide the majority of rumen undegraded protein, lysine appears to be limiting, while methionine is thought to be limiting for diets containing lower amounts of maize and supplemented with vegetable or animal proteins (Polan, Cummins, Sniffen, Muscato, Viciani, Crooker, Clark, Johnson, Otterby, Guillaume, Miller, Varga, Murray and Peirce-Sandner 1991, Schwab, Bozak, Whitehouse and Mesbah, 1992). Further studies in cows fed grass silage supplemented with cereal-based concentrates have implicated histidine (Kim, Choung and Chamberlain, 1999, Korhonen, Vanhatalo, Huhtanen and Varvikko, 2000, Vanhatalo, Huhtanen, Toivonen and Varvikko, 1999), rather than leucine (Huhtanen, Vanhatalo and Varvikko, 2002), methionine or lysine (Varvikko, Vanhatalo, Jalava and Huhtanen, 1999) as first limiting. Even when post-ruminal infusions of single AA have stimulated increases in milk protein, responses are generally confined to an increase in output rather than concentration (Table 3). In cases where infusions cause an imbalance in the supply of essential AA, milk protein content is generally depressed (Cant *et al.*, 2002, Choung and Chamberlain, 1992).

Rumen protected sources of methionine and lysine have been developed in an attempt to mimic responses attained using post-ruminal infusions. Milk production and composition responses to rumen protected methionine and lysine have been extensively reviewed (Robinson, 1996, Rulquin *et al.*, 1993, Sloan, 1997). Even though protected AA can stimulate improvements in milk protein content and secretion, responses are highly variable due to differences in the amount and profile of absorbed AA derived from the basal diet (Rulquin and Vérité, 1993). In a recent appraisal, Cant *et al.* (2002) concluded that milk protein responses to alterations in the supply of a single AA do not conform to expectations owing to transport rates of individual AA within the mammary gland being based on a threshold that is dictated to by physiological state, nutritional status and milk removal rate. This suggestion is consistent with larger milk protein responses being attained when the supply of the first limiting AA is increased using dietary protein supplements compared with post-ruminal infusions (Korhonen *et al.*, 2000, Korhonen *et al.*, 2002). It appears that greater improvements in milk protein secretion may be result from rumen-protected supplements containing a mixture of essential AA rather than a single limiting AA.

Responses to gluconeogenic substrates

High yielding dairy cows have a specific glucose requirement for lactose synthesis. The mammary gland accounts for proportionately between 0.60 and 0.85 of total glucose utilisation in lactating animals, most of which is used for lactose synthesis. Glucose absorption from the intestine of ruminant animals is limited and therefore most of the glucose released into the peripheral circulation is synthesised in the liver from propionate,

Table 3. Milk production responses to post-ruminal infusions of single amino acids.

	Infusion rate (g/day)					Significance [a]		Reference
						Linear	Quadratic	
Methionine	0	8	16	32				Guinard and Rulquin, 1995
Milk protein yield (g/day)	674	660	707	689				
Milk fat yield (g/day)	984	969	1003	1021				
Milk protein content (g/kg)	2.77	2.87	2.91	2.88		#		
Milk fat content (g/kg)	4.06	4.17	4.12	4.26				
Methionine	0	10	20	30	40			Varvikko *et al.*, 1999
Milk protein yield (g/day)	788	777	810	815	804			
Milk fat yield (g/day)	992	999	1037	1038	1064	***		
Milk protein content (g/kg)	31.8	31.7	32.4	32.1	32.0			
Milk fat content (g/kg)	39.9	40.5	41.2	40.7	42.1	*		
Lysine	0	9	27	63				Guinard and Rulquin, 1994
Milk protein yield (g/day)	670	702	698	683				
Milk fat yield (g/day)	949	972	908	993				
Milk protein content (g/kg)	31.0	31.4	32.0	31.3				
Milk fat content (g/kg)	43.5	43.5	41.9	45.4		*	*	
Lysine	0	15	30	45	60			Varvikko *et al.*, 1999
Milk protein yield (g/day)	702	710	709	704	694			
Milk fat yield (g/day)	919	951	954	912	918		#	
Milk protein content (g/kg)	32.0	32.3	32.0	32.2	31.7			
Milk fat content (g/kg)	41.9	43.2	43.1	41.8	42.1			

Table 3. continued

	Infusion rate (g/day)				*Significance* [a]		*Reference*
	0	2	4	6	*Linear*	*Quadratic*	
Histidine							Korhonen *et al.*, 2000
Milk protein yield (g/day)	861	877	907	919	**		
Milk fat yield (g/day)	1240	1167	1296	1177			
Milk protein content (g/kg)	3.19	3.13	3.22	3.20			
Milk fat content (g/kg)	4.60	4.16	4.60	4.09	*		

[a] Significance of linear and quadratic responses to infusions at $P < 0.10$, $P < 0.05$, $P < 0.01$ and $P < 0.001$ levels are indicated by #, *, ** and ***, respectively.

AA, glycerol, lactate and pyruvate (Brockman, 1993). Propionate is the major gluconeogenic substrate in ruminant species and accounts for proportionately between 0.46 and 0.55 of hepatic glucose release in lactating dairy cows (Seal and Reynolds, 1993). Alanine, aspartate, glutamate and glutamine are the major AA precursors of hepatic glucose production in lactating cattle (Black, Anand, Bruss, Brown and Nakagiri, 1990) under the regulatory control of insulin and glucagon. Under normal conditions proportionately 0.16 of hepatic glucose production is thought to arise from AA catabolism (Huntington, 1990).

Short-term studies using hyperinsulinemic-euglycaemic clamps and intravenous infusions of glucose and insulin over a four-day period have shown that increases in insulin concentration are associated with an increase in both milk protein content and yield (McGuire, Griinari, Dwyer and Bauman, 1995). Subsequent studies expanded on these observations and demonstrated that milk protein responses were enhanced yet further when insulin infusions were combined with abomasal infusions of casein (Griinari, McGuire, Dwyer, Bauman, Barbano and House, 1997) or casein and branched-chained AA (Mackle, Dwyer, Ingvartsen, Chouinard, Lynch, Barbano and Bauman, 1999, Mackle *et al.*, 2000). Insulin does not appear to enhance AA uptake by the mammary gland (Metcalf, Sutton, Cockburn, Napper and Beever, 1991, Tesseraud, Grizard, Makarski, Debras, Bayle and Champredon, 1992) but may act by inhibiting gluconeogenic and oxidative AA catabolism. Since increases in propionate or glucose stimulate pancreatic release of insulin, it is reasonable to assume that diets that promote rumen propionate production or increase glucose absorption would also stimulate higher rates of milk protein synthesis as a direct response to endocrine controls, sparing of AA from gluconeogenesis, or both.

Production of volatile fatty acids (VFA) in the rumen is the primary form in which energy yielding substrates enter the blood in ruminant animals. A substantial amount of VFA are metabolised during absorption from the rumen wall. Proportionately between 0.40-69, 0.30-0.78 and 0.08-0.66 of acetate, propionate and butyrate produced in the rumen are thought to enter portal blood (Seal and Reynolds, 1993). The majority of absorbed propionate and butyrate is metabolised in the liver and only acetate enters peripheral blood in appreciable amounts (Seal and Reynolds, 1993). Changes in the pattern of VFA absorbed from the rumen into portal blood can be induced through intra-ruminal infusions or changes in the diet. Intra-ruminal infusions of propionate typically increase milk protein synthesis but the magnitude of response is extremely variable (Thomas and Chamberlain, 1984). Positive effects on milk protein synthesis have in some cases been realised as an increase in both milk protein content and yield (Rook and Balch, 1961, Rook, Balch and Johnson, 1965) or more typically confined to higher milk protein output (Huhtanen, Blauwiekel and Saastamoinen, 1998, Hurtaud, Rulquin and Vérité, 1993, Miettinen and Huhtanen, 1996). Molar proportions of propionate in total VFA can be increased by the amount and type of concentrate supplements for diets based on grass hay (Robinson, 1996, Sutton, Broster, Schuller, Napper, Broster and Bines, 1988, Sutton, Morant, Bines, Napper and Givens, 1993, Thomas and Chamberlain, 1982) or replacing grass silage with maize silage (Fitzgerald and Murphy, 1999). For grass silage diets, rumen fermentation pattern is primarily determined by the extent of silage fermentation (Chamberlain and Choung, 1995, Keady and Mayne, 2001) and is generally resistant to manipulation using concentrate supplements (Huhtanen, 1998, Jaakkola and Huhtanen, 1993, Keady and Mayne, 2001, Thomas and Chamberlain, 1982). In these cases, molar proportions of propionate are more closely associated with silage lactic acid content (Martin, Chamberlain, Robertson and Hirst, 1994). Diets based on restrictively fermented grass silage are characterised by low molar proportions of glucogenic relative to lipogenic short chain FA and provide only small amounts of post-ruminal starch. Under these circumstances it is has been suggested that glucose supply may be limited for lactose synthesis leading to compromised milk protein synthesis due to a higher dependence on AA for gluconeogenesis (Huhtanen, 1998). This hypothesis has been recently been tested by examining milk production responses to dietary supplements of a gluconeogenic substrate, or following intravenous or post-ruminal infusions of glucose in cows fed diets based on restrictively fermented silage. Feeding supplements of propylene glycol with formic acid treated grass silage reduced milk protein content and output, but increased milk protein synthesis on comparable diets based on inoculant treated and untreated grass silages (Shingfield, Jaakkola and Huhtanen, 2002b). The lack of response with restrictively fermented silage was against expectations, since these diets had lower molar proportions of propionate in rumen VFA compared with the extensively fermented silages (Shingfield, Jaakkola and Huhtanen, 2002a).

Intravenous infusions of glucose have had variable effects on milk protein. At low levels, milk protein concentrations and output have been depressed, but have been increased at high rates of infusion (Table 4). Infusions of glucose in the abomasum have been shown to improve milk protein output in the absence of changes in milk protein content (Huhtanen *et al.*, 2002). In cases where glucose is also infused with limiting AA, either none (Kim, Choung and Chamberlain, 2000) or positive effects (Huhtanen *et al.*, 2002) on milk protein secretion have been reported, whilst intravenous infusions of histidine with glucose were found to have no beneficial effects on milk protein synthesis compared with histidine alone (Kim, Kim, Choung and Chamberlain, 2001).

Examination of milk production responses to post-ruminal infusions of glucose or starch provide a useful insight into the potential for improving milk protein synthesis with diets that encourage increases in glucose supply. Thomas and Chamberlain (1984) concluded that glucose infusions in cows fed diets based on grass hay or maize silage could be expected to increase milk protein yield, but reduce milk protein content. More recent studies examining milk production responses to intravenous glucose infusions or post-ruminal infusions of glucose and starch across a wider range of diets indicate that increases in glucose supply often stimulate marginal increases in milk protein output, but have only minor effects on milk protein concentrations (Table 4). It is less clear if these responses can be attained under practical feeding conditions, because diets formulated to enhance glucose supply would also alter the availability of other nutrients that is not the case under controlled experimental conditions.

Increasing the amount of dietary starch reaching the small intestine represents one nutritional approach for increasing glucose absorption in ruminant animals. It has been suggested that increases in the amount of starch digested in the small intestine could increase milk protein output through the sparing of AA from catabolism in the gut and liver (Nocek and Tamminga, 1991, Reynolds, Harmon and Cecava, 1994). However, this hypothesis has been questioned, since reductions in the catabolism of glutamine, glutamate and aspartate, that are relatively abundant in microbial protein and serve as the principal energy yielding amino acids for gut enterocytes, would not directly increase the supply of limiting AA (Reynolds, Sutton and Beever, 1997). Studies involving post-ruminal infusions of partially hydrolysed starch (Knowlton, Dawson, Glenn, Huntington and Erdman, 1998), maize or wheat starch (Reynolds, Cammell, Humphries, Beever, Sutton and Newbold, 2001) have shown that while increases in starch availability often increase milk protein output, responses are not realised as higher milk protein concentrations (Table 4). Reynolds *et al.* (2001) interpreted the lack of changes in milk protein content as being inconsistent with higher glucose absorption from the gut increasing AA availability to the mammary gland.

Based on an extensive evaluation of published data, Nocek and Tamminga (1991) concluded that there was little evidence to suggest that increases in post-ruminal starch digestion would improve milk production. While these conclusions are subject to criticism, because in most studies the site of starch digestion is confounded with energy intake (Reynolds, Sutton and Beever, 1997), more recent appraisals have concluded that shifting starch digestion towards the small intestine at the expense of the rumen often have more negative than positive effects on milk yield and composition (Huntington, 1997, Theurer, Huber, Delgado-Edorduy and Wanderley, 1999). Detrimental effects are thought

Table 4. Milk production responses to glucose and starch infusions

Infusate	Infusion site	Basal forage	Infusion (g/day)	Mean response per 100 g infusate [a]					Reference
				Milk	Milk protein		Milk fat		
				Yield (g/day)	Content (g/kg)	Output (g/day)	Content (g/kg)	Output (g/day)	
Glucose	Jugular vein	Grass silage	100	-100	-1.50	-37.0	1.50	32.0	Kim *et al.*, 2000
Glucose	Jugular vein	Grass silage	230	261	0.61	20.4	-0.30	6.1	Kim *et al.*, 2000
Glucose	Abomasum	Grass silage	250	320	0.12	9.6	-0.28	4.4	Huhtanen *et al.*, 2002
Glucose	Duodenum	Dehydrated maize	1500	-53	0.10	0.9	-0.24	-8.3	Lemosquet *et al.*, 1997
Glucose	Duodenum	Maize silage	500-1500	-13	0.04	1.8	-0.63	-25.0	Hurtaud *et al.*, 1998
Glucose	Duodenum	Grass silage	250-2000	219	-0.08	3.5	-0.35	-2.0	Hurtaud *et al.*, 2000
Glucose	Duodenum	Grass silage	750-2250	163	0.03	5.9	-0.17	-2.4	Hurtaud *et al.*, 2000
Starch [b]	Rumen	Lucerne silage	1500	140	-0.03	2.6	-0.10	1.1	Knowlton *et al.*, 1998
Starch [b]	Abomasum	Lucerne silage	1500	120	0.06	5.7	-0.03	3.1	Knowlton *et al.*, 1998
Maize starch	Duodenum	Grass silage	700-2100	126	0.01	4.7	-0.17	0.0	Reynolds *et al.*, 2001
Wheat starch	Duodenum	Dehydrated lucerne	1200	-67	0.01	-1.8	-0.08	-4.0	Reynolds *et al.*, 2001

[a] Responses calculated as the difference between treatment controls and infusion treatments and expressing the response per 100 g infusate. For studies where several various infusion levels were evaluated, responses were calculated as the mean across all infusion treatments.
[b] Refers to partially hydrolysed starch

to reflect reductions in total tract starch digestibility and associated decreases in microbial protein synthesis in the rumen.

Inclusion of starch in the diet has often been reported to increase the proportion of propionate in rumen VFA largely at the expense of acetate (Keady and Mayne, 2001, Overton, Cameron, Elliot, Clark and Nelson, 1995, Robinson, 1996, Sutton *et al.*, 1988, Sutton, Cammell, Phipps, Beever and Humphries, 2000). Propionate is the major gluconeogenic precursor in lactating dairy cows (Danfaer, Tetens and Agergaard, 1995, Seal and Reynolds, 1993), leading to considerable interest in manipulating dietary starch concentrations to effect changes in rumen fermentation pattern, and hence milk composition. Starch intakes can be manipulated by harvesting maize or cereal silages from crops at more advanced stages of maturity or through the replacement of fibrous with starch rich ingredients in concentrate supplements. Feeding maize silage harvested at dry matter contents of 280 and 330 g/kg have resulted in significantly higher milk protein yields compared with those harvested at 230 or 380 g DM/kg, but the effects were not directly related to the intake of maize starch (Phipps, Sutton, Beever and Jones, 2000). Similarly, ensiling whole crop wheat at two DM contents had no effect on milk protein content or yield despite substantial differences in the intake of wheat starch (Sutton, Phipps, Deaville, Jones and Humphries, 2002). Cereals are the predominant source of starch in ruminant diets while feeds such as sugar-beet pulp and citrus pulp are rich in digestible neutral detergent fibre. Often these ingredients have been used to examine the effect of dietary energy source on milk composition. Milk production responses to increases in starch intake on grass silage based diets have been disappointingly inconsistent. Replacing digestible fibre with starch has in some cases increased (e.g. Aston, Thomas, Daley and Sutton, 1994, Keady, Mayne and Marsden, 1998, Keady, Mayne, Fitzpatrick and Marsden, 1999, Thomas, Aston, Daley and Bass, 1986), or in others (e.g. Castle, Gill and Watson, 1981, Huhtanen, Jaakkola and Saarisalo, 1995, Mayne and Gordon, 1984, Sloan, Rowlinson and Armstrong, 1988) had no effect on milk protein content.

In an attempt to assess the effect of concentrate energy source on milk production and composition mean treatment values (n = 39) reported from 17 studies were subjected to meta-analysis using a mixed model that accounted for variations between experiments according to St Pierre (2001). While it is accepted that the comparison is rather limited, this approach does provide a useful insight into the possible outcomes arising from changes in dietary energy source. Based on derived regression equations (Figure 2) replacing fibre with starch in concentrate supplements resulted in 0.04 proportionate decreases in milk yield, but stimulated 0.02 and 0.15 proportionate increases in milk protein output and the ratio of protein to fat, respectively.

In recent studies where incremental amounts of concentrate fibre have been replaced with starch, milk protein concentrations have been increased irrespective of silage fermentation characteristics (Keady, Mayne and Marsden, 1998, Keady *et al.*, 1999). Beneficial effects were not associated with significant increases in the proportion of propionate in rumen VFA, and therefore (Keady and Mayne, 2001) attributed the positive effects on milk protein to increases in microbial protein supply. Whether these responses truly reflect changes in rumen fermentation pattern or beneficial effects on microbial protein synthesis remains unclear. Replacing high-moisture maize with citrus pulp in total mixed rations based on lucerne silage decreased milk protein content and reduced the proportion of propionate in rumen VFA (Broderick, Mertens and Simons, 2002), while replacing sugar beet pulp with barley had no effect on microbial protein supply in cattle fed grass silage (Huhtanen, 1988). In other studies, supplementing grass silage based diets with steam-flaked maize starch has increased EMPS and microbial protein supply (Van Vuuren, Klop, Van der Koelen and De Visser, 1999; Figure 4).

Responses to energy intake

There is a general consensus in the literature that energy intake is the major attribute of the diet influencing milk protein content. Based on data across a range of energy intakes (38 to 170 MJ/day), Emery (1978) estimated that milk protein content increased proportionately 0.015 per Mcal of additional NE_l intake, equivalent to 0.0022/MJ ME. Evaluation of 53 production trials also suggested that each additional MJ of ME intake elicited 0.003 proportionate increases in milk protein content (Spörndly, 1989). As Sutton (1989) noted, correlation coefficients describing the relationships between deviations from the mean for milk protein with those for energy intake for each treatment within individual experiments were consistent between both sets of data (r value 0.42) despite differences in cow breed and diet type. In assessing the positive association between milk protein content and secretion with energy intake, Coulon and Remond (1991) estimated that in early and mid-lactation cows each additional MJ of ME intake could be expected to result in respective 0.04 and 0.08 g/kg increases in milk protein content. While the relationship between energy intake and milk protein synthesis is widely accepted, it is clear that this only holds true when increases in ME are derived from non-lipid sources. Across a wide range of diets, milk protein concentrations have been found to be negatively associated with dietary ether extract content (Sporndly, 1989), such that lipid supplements typically cause a 1-4 g/kg reduction in milk protein content (Table 5). Often the negative effects have been attributed to increases in milk yield rather than reductions in milk protein output (DePeters and Cant, 1992). It is becoming increasingly clear that these decreases are not simply due to dilution, but reflect true physiological responses to

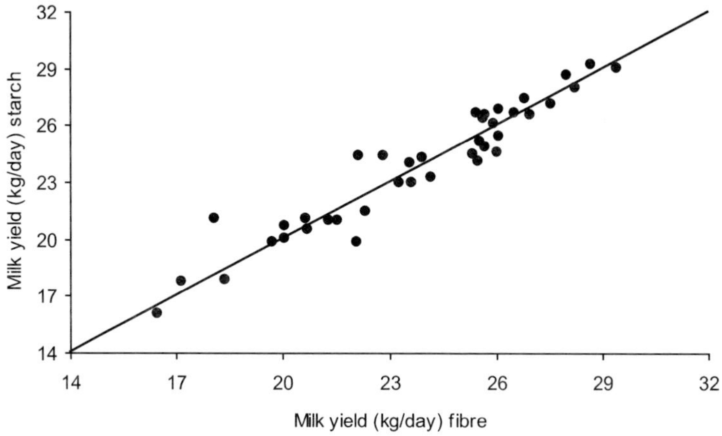

Figure 4. Effect of replacing digestible fibre (FIBRE) with starch (STARCH) in concentrate supplements on a) milk yield, b) milk protein yield and c) the ratio of milk protein to fat from grass silage based diets.

a) Milk yield

Line fitted represents the regression equation:
$Y = 0.96$ (s.e. 0.048) $x + 1.1$ (1.15) $n = 39$, $r^2 = 0.913$, $P < 0.001$

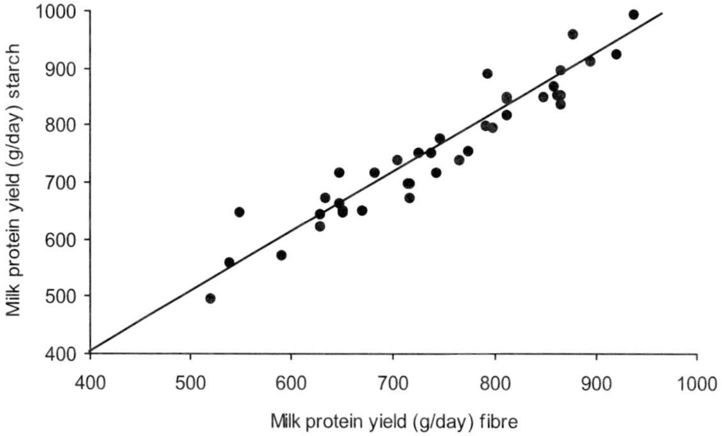

b) Milk protein yield

Line fitted represents the regression equation:
$Y = 1.02$ (s.e. 0.052) $x + 0.3$ (38.77) $n = 39$, $r^2 = 0.910$, $P < 0.001$

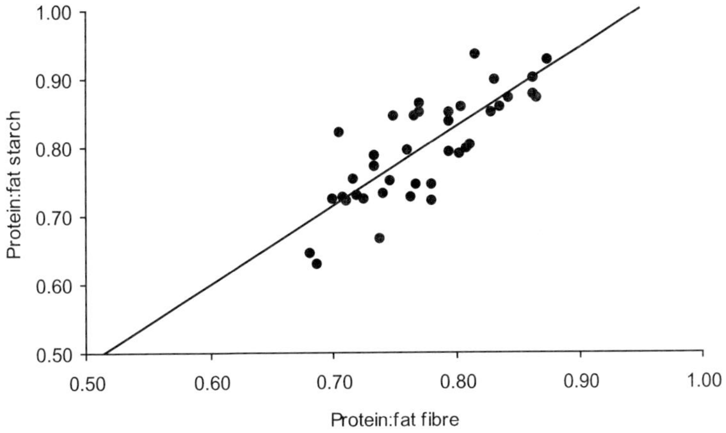

c) Milk protein:fat ratio

Line fitted represents the regression equation:

$Y = 1.15$ (s.e. 0.142) x - 0.09 (0.110) $n = 39$, $r^2 = 0.629$, $P < 0.001$

Data derived from studies where sugar beet pulp has been replaced by barley (Castle, Gill and Watson, 1981); (Chamberlain, Thomas, Wilson, Kassem and Robertson, 1984); (Mayne and Gordon, 1984); (Murphy, 1986); (Huhtanen *et al.*, 1993); (Huhtanen, 1987); (Dewhurst, Aston, Fisher, Evans, Dhanoa and McAllan, 1999); (Romney, Blunn, Sanderson and Leaver, 2000), ground wheat or sodium hydroxide treated whole wheat (O'Mara, Murphy and Rath, 1997), citrus pulp has been replaced with barley (Sloan *et al.*, 1988); sugar-beet pulp, wheat bran and barley fibre has been replaced with oats and barley (Huhtanen *et al.*, 1995); molassed sugar beet pulp and citrus pulp have been replaced with barley, wheat and maize gluten (Keady *et al.*, 1999, Keady *et al.*, 1998), unmolassed sugar beet pulp and extracted rice bran have been replaced with barley (Thomas *et al.*, 1986), sugar beet and citrus pulp or straw has been replaced with wheat feed, wheat and barley (Thomas and Robertson, 1987); wheat feed, molassed sugar beet pulp and citrus pulp have been replaced with barley and wheat (Phipps *et al.*, 1987), or alkali treated straw, unmolassed sugar beet pulp, distillers dark grains and dried grass were replaced with barley, wheat and cassava (Aston *et al.*, 1994).

lipid supplements (Garnsworthy, 1997, Wu and Huber, 1994). In an extensive evaluation of data from 49 studies, Wu and Huber (1994) concluded that the extent of decrease was largely independent of fat source, with the exception of fat prills. However, more recent studies have found no evidence that feeding flaked or prilled tallow of different saturation increase milk protein concentrations (Eastridge and Firkins, 2000).

Possible mechanisms underlying changes in milk protein content in response to fat supplements have been attributed to deficiencies in glucose supply, insulin resistance, improved energetic efficiency of milk production or reduced somatotrophin production (Wu and Huber, 1994). Of these, limitations in glucose supply appear to be the most plausible. It has been argued that glucose could become more limiting due to reductions in propionate production and microbial protein synthesis when fat replaces starch in the diet, or due to increased glucose requirements for triacylglyceride transport in the gut mucosa and lactose synthesis when fat stimulates an increase in milk yield (Garnsworthy, 1997). In support of this hypothesis, lactose supplements were found to partially overcome depressions in milk protein content when calcium salts of palm oil FA replaced cereals in the diet (Garnsworthy, 1996). Further studies indicated that increases in dietary rumen undegradable protein were capable of maintaining milk protein concentrations when milk yield was increased using rumen protected fat, while a combination of protected rapeseed and lactose proved to be even more effective (Garnsworthy, 1997).

In addition to fat supplements, energy intake can be increased using concentrate supplements or replacing grass silage with forages of higher intake potential and/or energy content. Increases in concentrate supplementation enhance total DM intake, but reduce forage DM intake to a variable extent (Thomas, 1987). As a result, improvements in energy intake with concentrate supplements are often lower than expected due to negative associative effects on digestion (Huhtanen, 1998). Increasing the proportion of concentrate supplements in the diet would be expected to increase milk protein content since positive associations reported with energy intake (Emery, 1978, Spörndly, 1989) are simply a reflection of reductions in dietary forage to concentrate ratios.

Data from recent experiments indicate that concentrate supplementation of grass silage based diets increase milk protein content to a variable extent (Table 6). Some of the variation in response may reflect differences in DM intake arising from variable forage substitution rates, that are known to be affected by fermentation characteristics and digestibility of ensiled forages, composition of concentrate supplements (Thomas, 1987) and forage type (Dewhurst, Wadhwa, Borgida and Fisher, 2001a, Faverdin, Dulphy, Coulon, Vérité, Garel, Rouel and Marquis, 1991).

Table 5. Milk production responses to dietary lipid supplements

Lipid	Basal forage	Inclusion (g/kg DM)	Mean response [a]					Reference
			Milk	Milk protein		Milk fat		
			Yield (kg/day)	Content (g/kg)	Output (g/day)	Content (g/kg)	Output (g/day)	
Rapeseed oil	Maize	35	-1.9	-1.7	-112	0.0	-56	Jenkins, 1998
Rapeseed oil	Maize silage	33	0.8	-0.7	3	-2.8	-80	Loor *et al.*, 2002
Fish oil	Maize silage	17	1.5	-0.9	16	-13.3	-300	Chilliard and Doreau, 1997
Fish oil	Grass silage	16	0.4	-3.0	-35	-10.9	-167	Offer *et al.*, 1999
Fish oil	Maize silage/Lucerne	30	-4.3	0.0	-136	-6.7	-311	Donovan *et al.*, 2000
Fish oil	Grass silage	31	3.2	-3.8	7	-15.0	-250	Keady *et al.*, 2000
Fish oil	Grass/maize silage	37	-4.5	-2.4	-198	-10.0	-358	Ahnadi *et al.*, 2002
Partially hydrogenated vegetable shortening	Maize silage	37	-3.2	-0.6	-127	-1.0	-134	Kalscheur *et al.*, 1997
Linseed oil	Grass silage	16	1.8	-1.1	41	-0.8	69	Offer *et al.*, 1999
Linseed oil	Grass silage	27	0.6	-0.7	2	0.7	34	Shingfield *et al.*, unpublished
Soyabean oil	Maize silage	35	0.4	-0.1	10	-6.7	-189	Jenkins *et al.*, 1996
Soyabean oil	Grass silage	27	1.8	-1.2	42	0.2	82	Shingfield *et al.*, unpublished
Sunflower oil	Maize silage	37	-0.8	-1.2	-59	-3.0	-104	Kalscheur *et al.*, 1997

Table 5. continued

Lipid	*Basal forage*	*Inclusion (g/kg DM)*	*Mean response* [a]					*Reference*
			Milk	*Milk protein*		*Milk fat*		
			Yield (kg/day)	*Content (g/kg)*	*Output (g/day)*	*Content (g/kg)*	*Output (g/day)*	
Sunflower oil	Grass silage	50	2.0	-2.3	24	-3.1	38	Shingfield *et al.*, unpublished
Tallow	Maize silage	40	-4.2	0.9	-101	-3.0	-253	Onetti *et al.*, 2001
Tallow	Maize silage	30						
White grease	Maize silage	40	-4.2	1.1	-94	-4.5	-310	Onetti *et al.*, 2001
Protected lipids								
Butylsoyamide [b]	Maize silage	35	-1.7	-0.8	-78	-0.7	-74	Jenkins *et al.*, 1996
Canolamide [c]	Maize silage	33	-4.9	-1.7	-206	-2.7	-263	Loor *et al.*, 2002b
Ca-salts of linseed oil	Grass/maize silage	40	2.9	-1.9	0	-4.9	-110	Chouinard, Girard and Brisson, 1998
Ca-salts of palm oil	Maize silage	40	1.2	-1.0	13	-10.1 [d]	-162 [d]	Enjalbert *et al.*, 1997
Ca-salts of rapeseed oil	Maize silage	40	2.0	2.0	102	-0.6 [d]	76 [d]	Enjalbert *et al.*, 1997
Ca-salts of rapeseed oil	Grass/maize silage	40	0.3	-1.1	40	-13.8	-400	Chouinard, Girard and Brisson, 1998
Ca-salts of rapeseed oil	Grass silage	40	2.1	-1.6	30	-2.0	20	Kowalski, Pisulewski and Spanghero, 1999
Ca-salts of soyabean oil	Grass/maize silage	40	1.1	-2.0	-20	-10.7	-320	Chouinard, Girard and Brisson, 1998

Table 5. continued

Lipid	Basal forage	Inclusion (g/kg DM)	Mean response [a]					Reference
			Milk	Milk protein		Milk fat		
			Yield (kg/day)	Content (g/kg)	Output (g/day)	Content (g/kg)	Output (g/day)	
Oleamide [e]	Maize silage	35	-1.9	1.4	-26	-4.7	-187	Jenkins, 1998
Protected fish oil [f]	Grass/maize silage	30	-1.2	-4.6	-135	-15.6	-358	Ahnadi *et al.*, 2002

[a] Responses calculated as the difference between treatment controls and lipid supplemented diets.
[b] Prepared by reacting soyabean oil with butylamine.
[c] Prepared by reacting rapeseed oil with ethanolamide.
[d] Calculated assuming fatty acids were secreted as triglycerides and accounted for proportionately 0.90 of milk fat triacylglycerides.
[e] Prepared by reacting oleic acid with ammonia.
[f] Encapsulated fish oil in a glutaraldehyde-treated protein matrix.

Milk production responses to concentrate supplements determined in relatively short-term feeding studies have been confirmed in a recent long-term study performed across three lactations (Kennedy, Dillon, Faverdin, Delaby, Buckley and Rath, 2002). More intensive concentrate feeding was associated with a significant increase in milk protein content, irrespective of genetic merit. An earlier study examining milk production responses of medium and high genetic merit animals across a wide range in concentrate supplement levels (proportionately 0.37-0.70 of total diet DM) for a shorter period of time also noted comparable changes in milk protein content for both genotypes (Ferris, Gordon, Patterson, Mayne and Kilpatrick, 1999). Feeding more concentrate supplements can be used to increase milk protein content irrespective of animal genetic merit (Ferris *et al.*, 1999) or the nutritive value of grass silage (Ferris, Gordon, Patterson, Kilpatrick, Mayne and McCoy, 2001), but the benefits become progressively reduced at high levels (Figure 5).

In spite of a lower digestibility maize silage has a higher intake and milk production potential than grass silage (Fitzgerald and Murphy, 1999, O'Mara, Murphy and Rath, 1998). Development of early maturing varieties has increased the opportunity for growing maize in marginal areas within Northern Europe. In regions that are unable to support maize production, there has been considerable interest in whole-crop cereals as an alternative or complementary forage for grass silage based milk productions systems. This interest stems from high DM yields per hectare of whole crop cereals and the increased frequency of low rainfall during critical periods that compromise grass growth. A number of studies have examined milk production responses to partial or complete replacement of grass silage with maize or whole-crop cereal silages. Inclusion of whole-crop cereal silages increase DM intake, but the effects on milk production and composition are generally small and insignificant (Table 7). Based on two experiments, Leaver and Hill (1995) concluded that ensiled or urea treated whole-crop wheat could replace proportionately 0.40 of grass silage without adversely affecting milk production. Further studies have shown that milk production remains unaffected at higher inclusion levels (Sutton, Abdalla, Phipps, Cammell and Humphries, 1997, Sutton, Cammell, Beever, Humphries and Phipps, 1998). In contrast, replacing grass with maize silage has consistently increased milk production and milk protein content (Table 7). Positive effects on milk protein concentration have been attained even when maize silage has contained relatively low amounts of starch (Fitzgerald and Murphy, 1999, O'Mara, Murphy and Rath, 1998, Phipps *et al.*, 2000). It is a popular perception that improvements in milk protein content associated with feeding maize silage are related to higher intakes of energy and the amount of starch available for absorption from the small intestine. However, this explanation ignores changes in rumen fermentation and alterations in post-absorptive metabolic and endocrine

Table 6. Milk production responses to increases in concentrate supplementation

Basal forage	Range in supplement offered (kg/day)	Mean response per kg concentrate DM intake [a]					Reference
		Milk	Milk protein		Milk fat		
		Yield (kg/day)	Content (g/kg)	Output (g/day)	Content (g/kg)	Output (g/day)	
Grass silage	3 - 6	1.6	0.30	61.0	0.23	70.3	Sutton *et al.*, 1994
Grass silage	2 - 4	0.61	0.50	25.5	0.39	31.1	Agnew *et al.*, 1996
Grass silage	4 - 6	1.12	0.35	37.7	-0.71	29.4	
Grass silage	6 - 8	0.59	0.82	34.3	-1.00	0.63	
Grass silage	2 - 8	0.77	0.56	32.4	-0.42	20.6	
Grass silage	2 – 4	1.93	-0.06	55.2	1.32	94.3	Keady and Murphy, 1996
Grass silage	4 – 6	1.11	0.58	38.2	0.46	46.8	
Grass silage	2 – 6	1.52	0.26	46.7	0.89	70.6	
Grass silage	4 - 6	0.82	0.12	29.4	0.06	35.3	Fitzgerald and Murphy, 1999
Grass silage	6 – 8	0.95	0.42	36.8	-0.53	21.1	
Grass silage	4 – 8	0.89	0.28	33.3	-0.25	27.8	
Grass silage	7 – 10	0.51	0.31	24.8	-0.28	19.7	Rinne *et al.*, 1999b
Grass silage	7 – 10	0.72	0.39	35.6	0.00	33.4	Shingfield *et al.*, 2002b
Maize silage	4 - 6	0.41	0.65	29.4	-0.24	17.7	Fitzgerald and Murphy, 1999
Maize silage	6 - 8	0.47	0.35	23.5	0.94	47.1	
Maize silage	4 - 8	0.44	0.50	26.5	0.35	32.4	

[a] Responses calculated as the difference between treatment controls and supplemented diets and expressing the response on a kg concentrate DM intake basis.

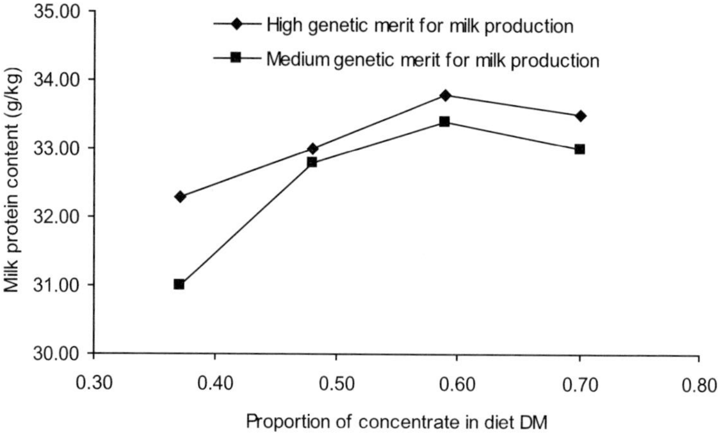

a) Genotype

Figure 5. Effect of genotype and nutritive value of grass silage on milk protein content responses to increases in concentrate supplementation

Data derived from (Ferris *et al.*, 1999).

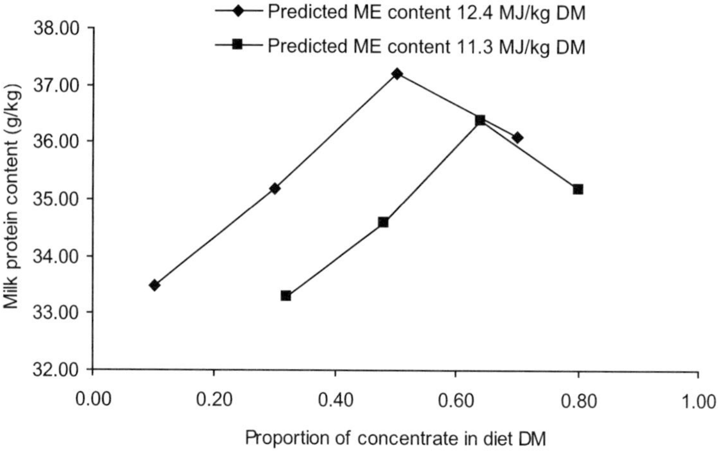

b) Nutritive value

Data derived from (Ferris et al., 2001).

status (Reynolds, Sutton and Beever, 1997). Replacing grass silage with maize silage would be expected to increase the amount of microbial AA available for absorption, since microbial protein synthesis is essentially a function of organic matter intake (Shingfield, 2000) and is energetically more efficient for maize than grass silage based diets (Givens and Rulquin, 2002). Furthermore, these changes increase molar propionate proportions in rumen VFA (Fitzgerald and Murphy, 1999), whilst post-ruminal infusions of maize or wheat starch have not stimulated appreciable increases in milk protein content (Reynolds *et al.*, 2001). It appears that at least part of the increase in milk protein content associated with feeding maize silage may be explained by improvements in AA and gluconeogenic precursor supply.

Milk fat

Milk fat content and FA composition can be significantly altered through nutrition offering the opportunity to respond to market forces and human health recommendations. The impact of nutrition on fat content and composition has been extensively reviewed (Ashes, Gulati and Scott, 1997, Chilliard, 1993, Grummer, 1991, Jensen, 2002, Kennelly, 1996, Palmquist and Jenkins, 1980, Palmquist, Beaulieu and Barbano, 1993, Sutton, 1989). Following the introduction of milk quotas within the EU in 1984, manipulation of milk fat has become increasingly important. Even though milk payment schemes stipulate a minimum fat content, enforced by financial penalties, there is still scope for reducing fat content and producing more milk within a given quota. In addition, there is also the potential for developing nutritional strategies for altering milk FA composition in line with human health recommendations and consumer requirements. In assessing the ability to add value to milk and dairy products, Kennelly (1996) concluded that the optimal FA profile of milk fat is a moving target. Unfortunately there are no universal guidelines on the ideal FA profile of milk with respect to human health. In order to provide a definition the Wisconsin Milk Marketing Board sought the advice of industry and scientists (O'Donnell, 1989), who concluded that milk fat should ideally contain less than 10 % polyunsaturated FA (PUFA), no more than 8 % saturated FA and 82 % of monounsaturated FA (MUFA). However, such changes in liquid milk supplies are not possible using current technology and feeding practices, or likely to be achieved in the foreseeable future. Furthermore, there is an increasing body of evidence to support the view that an acceptable FA profile may not warrant such extreme changes (Kennelly, 1996).

Lipids in milk are primarily in the form of triacylglycerides (98%) with phospholipids and sterols accounting for 1.0 and 0.5 % of total lipids, respectively. Bovine milk is extremely complex and contains about 400 FA, a large proportion of which are derived from lipid metabolism in

Table 7. Intake and milk production responses to replacement of grass silage with maize or whole crop-cereal silage

Forage	Inclusion (g/kg forage DM)	DM intake (kg/day)	Mean response [a]					Reference
			Milk	Milk protein		Milk fat		
			Yield (kg/day)	Content (g/kg)	Output (g/day)	Content (g/kg)	Output (g/day)	
Fermented-whole crop wheat	330	0.8	-0.6	-0.3	-40	-1.2	-70	Leaver and Hill, 1995
	400	1.7	0.7	0.0	20	0.1	30	
	330	1.3	1.2	0.9	50	0.0	60	Phipps *et al.*, 1987
Urea treated whole-crop wheat [b]	330	0.4	-0.9	-0.6	-50	-0.9	-70	Leaver and Hill, 1995
	333	1.1	-0.3	0.9	3	2.0	25	Sutton *et al.*, 1997
	667	1.5	1.1	1.5	62	-0.5	34	
	667	2.4	1.2	0.4	46	0.7	84	Sutton *et al.*, 1998
Urea treated whole-crop wheat [c]	330	0.8	-0.1	0.0	-10	-0.5	-20	Leaver and Hill, 1995
	400	2.2	1.6	-0.1	40	-0.6	50	
	330	0.9	1.0	0.9	60	0.4	50	Phipps *et al.*, 1987
	333	1.0	0.4	1.1	30	2.1	57	Sutton *et al.*, 1997
	667	1.4	1.5	1.5	74	-1.2	38	
	1000	0.9	-0.2	1.3	14	-0.1	-15	
	333	1.8	1.2	0.2	44	0.7	78	Sutton *et al.*, 1998
	667	1.9	0.8	1.4	53	3.1	104	
Maize silage DM 354 [d]	330	1.3	3.4	1.3	160	0.1	150	Phipps *et al.*, 1987
	750	3.2	4.6	2.0	210	-1.1	170	

Table 7. Continued

Forage	Inclusion (g/kg forage DM)	DM intake (kg/day)	Mean response [a]					Reference
			Milk Yield (kg/day)	Milk protein Content (g/kg)	Milk protein Output (g/day)	Milk fat Content (g/kg)	Milk fat Output (g/day)	
DM 257	333	0.9	1.6	0.4	60	-1.0	30	O'Mara *et al.*, 1998
	667	1.6	1.7	1.0	80	-0.1	50	
	1000	1.9	1.3	0.3	50	-0.3	30	
DM 226	750	1.7	1.4	1.8	90	0.8	80	Phipps *et al.*, 2000
DM 290	750	4.1	4.7	2.1	197	-1.6	149	
DM 302	750	3.9	5.0	1.3	192	-3.2	112	
DM 390	750	3.6	2.8	1.3	122	-0.4	109	
DM 339	1000	4.3	-0.7	3.5	20	7.0	108	Mulligan *et al.*, 2002

[a] Responses calculated as the difference between treatment controls and supplemented diets.
[b] Urea applied at a rate of 20 g/kg DM
[c] Urea applied at a rate of 40 g/kg DM
[d] DM: dry matter content expressed as g/kg fresh weight.

the rumen (Jensen, 2002). Substrates for *de novo* synthesis are derived from ruminal fibre digestion and dietary lipids supply preformed FA for direct incorporation into milk fat (Figure 2). Microbial synthesis of branched and odd-chained number FA in the rumen and absorption of biohydrogenation intermediates also contribute to the diversity of FA secreted in milk fat. Under typical conditions, about half of the FA in milk are synthesised *de novo*, 40 to 45 % originate from fat in the diet, and less than 10 % are derived from mobilisation of adipose tissue (Palmquist and Jenkins, 1980). However, nutrition can substantially alter the balance between mammary *de novo* FA synthesis and uptake of preformed FA (Kennelly, 1996).

Lipid metabolism in the rumen

It is well established that ruminant lipids contain higher levels of saturated FA compared with ingested dietary lipids owing to extensive biohydrogenation of unsaturated FA in the rumen. On entering the rumen dietary lipids are exposed to microbial lipases that result in the release of NEFA. The FA liberated during hydrolysis are adsorbed onto feed particles and subjected to biohydrogenation or directly incorporated into bacterial lipids (Demeyer and Doreau, 1999). *Butyrivibrio fibrisolvens* was the first rumen bacteria identified as being capable of biohydrogenation (Polan, McNeill and Tove, 1964). Further studies indicated that a free carboxyl group was an absolute requirement for biohydrogenation of NEFA (Kepler, Hirons, McNeill and Tove, 1966). Following these observations, a number of bacteria have been identified as being capable of performing certain steps of the biohydrogenation process, and have been classified based on the profile of biohydrogenation intermediates produced. The most widely used scheme is that proposed by Kemp and Lander (1984) which assigns bacteria into two groups, A and B. Bacteria of group A are thought to biohydrogenate PUFA to *trans*-11 $C_{18:1}$, while group B bacteria convert $C_{18:1}$ FA to $C_{18:0}$ (Figure 6).

It was first thought that biohydrogenation of $C_{18:2}$ (n-6) and $C_{18:3}$ (n-3) simply involved the addition of hydrogen atoms. Wilde and Dawson (1966) were the first to demonstrated that biohydrogenation was more involved, following the production of a *cis*/*trans* intermediate during incubations of $^{14}C_{18:3}$ (n-3) with ovine rumen contents. This FA intermediate was identified as *cis*-9, *trans*-11, *cis*-15- $C_{18:3}$ (Kemp and Dawson, 1968). Similarly, the first step of $C_{18:2}$ (n-6) biohydrogenation also results in the formation of a conjugated FA, *cis*-9, *trans*-11- $C_{18:2}$ (Kepler *et al.*, 1966).

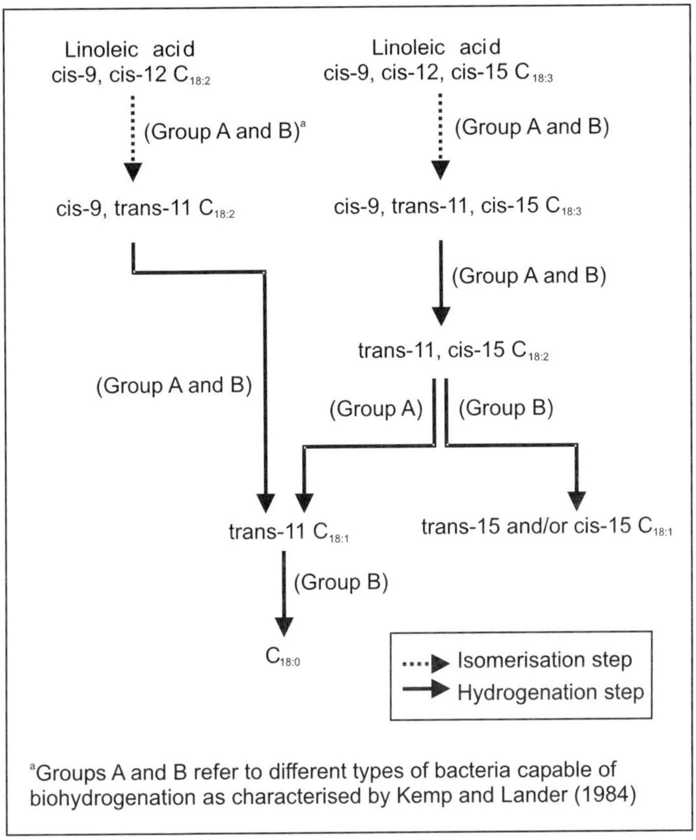

Figure 6. Pathways of ruminal biohydrogenation of polyunsaturated fatty acids (adapted from Harfoot and Hazlewood, 1997)

Based on established metabolic pathways (Figure 6), biohydrogenation of $C_{18:2}$ (n-6) and $C_{18:3}$ (n-3) results in the formation of a common intermediate *trans*-11 $C_{18:1}$. Positional isomers are possible, but under most conditions *trans*-11 $C_{18:1}$ is quantitatively the most important (Demeyer and Doreau, 1999). Eleven additional *trans* $C_{18:1}$ isomers can be produced, but only in small amounts through the activities of specific bacterial populations (Keeney, 1970). Only group-B bacteria can hydrogenate *cis* or *trans* $C_{18:1}$, indicating that biohydrogenation of $C_{18:2}$ (n-6) and $C_{18:3}$ (n-3) to $C_{18:0}$ requires both group A and B bacteria. The final reduction appears to be the rate limiting step, and therefore *trans* $C_{18:1}$ biohydrogenation intermediates can accumulate in the rumen (Keeney, 1970).

More recent studies have identified a rumen bacterium (*Megasphaera elsdenii YJ-4*) that is capable of converting $C_{18:2}$ (n-6) to *trans*-10, *cis*-12 $C_{18:2}$ (Kim, Liu, Rychlik and Russell, 2002). Even though *Butyrivibrio fibrisolvens* only expresses a *cis*-12, *trans*-11 isomerase it can hydrogenate *trans*-10, *cis*-12 $C_{18:2}$ to *trans*-10 $C_{18:1}$ in pure culture (Kepler *et al.*, 1966). *In vitro* studies have also shown that incubation of *cis*-9 $C_{18:1}$ (Mosley, Powell, Riley and Jenkins, 2002) or *trans*-9 $C_{18:1}$ (Proell, Mosley, Powell and Jenkins, 2002) results in the production of a wide range of *trans* $C_{18:1}$ isomers with double bonds in positions Δ-6 to Δ-16. Measurements of the flow of FA entering the omasal canal (Shingfield, Ahvenjärvi, Toivonen, Ärölä, Nurmela, Huhtanen and Griinari, 2003a) or duodenum (Duckett *et al.*, 2002, Piperova *et al.*, 2002) have confirmed this is also the case *in vivo*. The reasons for this are unclear, but one explanation is that rumen bacteria express several specific *cis*, *trans* isomerases, or alternatively positional *trans* $C_{18:1}$ isomers arise due to double bond migration (Griinari and Bauman, 1999).

Harfoot, Noble and Moore (1973) examined the rate of $C_{18:2}$ (n-6) biohydrogenation in different fractions of rumen fluid and showed that the vast majority of activity was associated with food particles. However, the role of food particles is less clear. It has been suggested that these particles are important to absorption of unsaturated FA by rumen bacteria (Harfoot, 1981). In support of this, Bauchart, Legay-Carmier, Doreau and Gaillard (1990) found that the FA content of surfacing-adhering-bacteria was twice that of liquid-associated bacteria.

In addition to lipids, other components of the diet also affect the rate and extent of biohydrogenation. Low-forage diets are known to be associated with reduced ruminal biohydrogenation (Latham, Storry and Sharpe, 1972) due to lowered ruminal lipolysis and reduced prevalence of *Butyrivibrio fibrisolvens*. Gerson, John and King (1985) found that adding fermentable carbohydrate to the diet did not inhibit hydrolysis or biohydrogenation. However, replacing fibre with fermentable carbohydrate resulted in a decrease in the rates of lipolysis and biohydrogenation, while higher amounts of dietary nitrogen increase these parameters (Gerson, John and Sinclair, 1983).

FA available for absorption are also derived from rumen microbes, primarily in the form of structural lipids. Bacterial and protozoal lipids make a considerable contribution to the total flow of lipid into the duodenum (Garton, 1977). Based on an extensive evaluation of the relationship between FA intake and the flow of FA in the duodenum, Doreau and Ferlay (1994) estimated the extent of microbial lipid synthesis as 9 g/kg DM intake.

Bacterial lipids originate from dietary FA and *de novo* synthesis. The contribution of exogenous and endogenous sources is dependent on dietary lipid content and bacterial species residing in the rumen (Harfoot and Hazlewood, 1997). PUFA are not commonly synthesised by rumen bacteria, and appear to arise from uptake of dietary FA (Jenkins, 1993). Branched-chain FA unique to ruminant lipids, are derived from rumen microbes (Harfoot and Hazlewood, 1997), as a result of chain elongation of precursors produced during the metabolism of branched-chain AA (Garton, 1977).

FA entering the duodenum are mainly adsorbed onto feed particles and bacteria. About 80 % of lipids in ruminal digesta are in form of NEFA, intimately associated with the particulate matter (Garton, 1977). The total amount of lipid entering the duodenum often exceeds ingestion due to microbial synthesis. On high forage diets, the flow of lipids entering the duodenum can exceed proportionately 0.40 of dietary intake (Sutton, Storry and Nicholson, 1970). Inclusion of dietary lipid supplements can result in higher, similar or lower post-ruminal flows relative to FA intake, due to the effects on microbial lipid synthesis (Demeyer and Doreau, 1999). Endogenous lipases do not play a significant role in the ruminant small intestine except when rumen protected lipids are fed (Garton, 1977). Digestive juices desorb FA and solubilise them into a micellar solution, that disperses FA into the liquid phase, and away from the solid material. Mucosal cells in the jejuneum absorb the micellar solution and the FA are esterified to triacylglycerides (Garton, 1977). These are then packaged within chylomicrons and VLDL (Demeyer and Doreau, 1999). After entering the lymphatic system lipoproteins and chylomicrons are transported to the circulatory system (Noble, 1981). Lipid is transported in plasma in the form of lipoproteins, primarily as cholesterol esters and phospholipid fractions, and to a much lesser extent triacylglycerides, NEFA and free cholesterol (Christie, 1981). The majority of FA entering the circulatory system are saturated. Small amounts of unsaturated FA that escape biohydrogenation are preferentially esterified into cholesterol esters and phospholipid fractions, mainly within HDL. HDL fractions are slowly turned over, unlike triacylglycerides and NEFA, which are turned over much faster and supply FA to other tissues such as the mammary gland (Noble, 1981).

Physiological factors

Breed is known to influence the concentration of the major constituents in milk. For example, mean milk fat content has been shown to be proportionately 0.19 (White, Bertrand, Wade, Washburn, Green and Jenkins, 2001) and 0.30 (Drackley, Beaulieu and Elliott, 2001) higher for Jersey than Holstein cows fed the same diet. In addition to fat content, breed also influences milk FA composition. On similar diets, concentrations of $C_{16:1}$, $C_{18:1}$ and CLA are higher and $C_{6:0}$, $C_{8:0}$, $C_{10:0}$, $C_{12:0}$ and $C_{14:0}$ content is lower for Holstein than Jersey dairy cows (White *et al.*, 2001). Comparison of responses of Holstein and Jersey cows to lipid supplements and the proportion of structural carbohydrates also indicated similar breed effects (Drackley, Beaulieu and Elliott, 2001). Higher levels of $C_{16:1}$, $C_{18:1}$ and CLA under the same dietary conditions are consistent with the view that the activity of Δ^9-desaturase is higher in Holstein than Jersey mammary tissue (Beaulieu and Palmquist, 1995), while the lower concentrations of short and medium chain FA suggest a lower proportion of FA secreted in Holstein milk are synthesised *de novo*.

In order to assess the impact of nutrition on milk fat content and composition it is essential that variation in genetic merit is taken into account. It is also important to recognise milk fat concentrations change with stage of lactation in much the same manner as milk protein. Tamminga (2001) noted for Holstein-Friesian cows, that milk fat content at the start of lactation was around 44 g/kg, decreased to about 40 g/kg after 2 months, and gradually increased to 48 g/kg at 300 days postpartum.

Nutrition has a greater effect on milk FA composition in early compared with mid to late lactation cows, in spite of the dilution of dietary FA with those mobilised from adipose tissue (Chilliard, 1993, Grummer, 1991). Early studies demonstrated that the transfer efficiency of intravenously infused labelled triacylglycerides to milk declined from 30% in early lactation to 5% in late lactation (Storry, 1981). Changes in apparent transfer efficiencies have been attributed to a higher proportion of absorbed FA being partitioned towards the mammary gland during negative energy balance, an effect that declines as lactation progresses (Grummer, 1991, Storry, 1981). Irrespective of diet, the proportion of $C_{4:0}$ to $C_{12:0}$ fatty acids in milk fat was lower in early lactation (< 30 days in milk) than mid (120 days) or late (210 days) lactation (Auldist, Walsh and Thomson, 1998). Such responses probably reflect the greater contribution of mobilised adipose tissue to mammary FA supply during early lactation.

Responses to amino acids

Numerous studies have attempted to establish the relative deficiencies of AA with respect to milk protein output. Even though the primary objective has been to establish the rate limiting AA for milk protein synthesis, these experiments have also demonstrated some interesting effects on milk fat content (Table 3). Post-ruminal infusions of single AA have variable effects on milk fat content, that possibly reflect AA requirements for milk protein synthesis, since an imbalance of essential AA tend to increase milk fat (Cant *et al.*, 2002, Choung and Chamberlain, 1992).

Responses to gluconeogenic substrates

Following the interest in increasing milk protein through the manipulation of dietary starch content, data has also become available on milk fat responses. In general, post-ruminal infusions of glucose or starch result in marginal decreases in milk fat content, that are often compensated for by increases in milk yield (Table 4). Only one study involving intravenous glucose infusions elicited positive effects on milk fat content and secretion (Kim, Choung and Chamberlain, 2000). It is perhaps not surprising that milk fat does not respond to increases in post-ruminal gluconeogenic supply, because rumen fermentation patterns and biohydrogenation of dietary FA remain unchanged. Even when starch has been infused in the rumen no effects on milk fat content or secretion have been observed (Knowlton *et al.*, 1998).

Responses to energy intake

Lipid supplements used to increase dietary energy content have variable effects on milk fat content (Table 5). Changes are dependent on lipid inclusion rate, degree of unsaturation and physical form (Sutton, 1989). Feeding fat supplements often reduces milk fat content, as a result of negative effects on ruminal OM digestion associated with decreases in intake and also changes in ruminal biohydrogenation. Of the responses reported in 28 comparisons (Table 5), lipid supplementation increased milk fat yield in six cases, while milk fat content was increased in only two studies. The largest increase in milk fat secretion was attained in cows fed 18 kg DM of grass silage based diets supplemented with 500 g/day of soyabean oil (Shingfield *et al.*, unpublished). The most consistent effect on milk fat content is the decrease with fish oil supplements. In general, inclusion of plant oils appears to have positive effects on milk fat output in animals fed grass silage based diets, but negative effects for maize based diets. The reasons for such differences are unclear, but may reflect the higher starch and lower NDF content of maize compared with grass and/or differences in ruminal biohydrogenation of forages rich in $C_{18:2}$ (n-6) and $C_{18:3}$ (n-3). Clearly the nature of the basal diet is an important determinant of milk fat responses to lipid supplements.

Various technological approaches have been developed to protect lipids from metabolism in the rumen, that include encapsulation of oils and oilseeds with a formaldehyde casein complex, calcium salts of FA or fatty acyl amides (Ashes, Gulati and Scott, 1997, Doreau and Ferlay, 1994). These products have primarily been developed to overcome the negative effects of feeding high levels of lipid supplements on animal performance (Mansbridge and Blake, 1997). In recent studies, feeding rumen protected lipids have decreased milk fat content, responses that were often associated with decreased milk fat output (Table 5), indicating that most supplements are only partially protected from lipolysis and biohydrogenation in the rumen. In summarising responses to a wide range of lipid supplements, Chilliard (1993) noted that only protected (encapsulated) tallow significantly increased milk fat content (mean 4.6 g/kg), and plant oils caused the largest depressions (mean -2.8 g/kg). Responses to protected tallow were found to be linear for intakes of 1.5

kg/day and in some cases exceeded 10 g/kg. Feeding oilseeds, particularly after heat-treatment are thought to offer natural protection from ruminal biohydrogenation (Doreau and Ferlay, 1994, Grummer, 1991). Compared with rapeseed meal, supplements of whole rapeseeds have depressed intake and milk yield, but the effects on milk fat content, secretion or FA composition are relatively minor (Delbecchi, Ahnadi, Kennelly and Lacasse, 2001).

Dietary inclusion of lipids is the most common nutritional means for manipulating milk FA composition. However, both the type and source of fat influences the extent of changes that can be achieved (Table 8). Supplements of plant oils or oilseeds reduce short and medium chain FA and increase long-chain FA in milk (Grummer, 1991, Mansbridge and Blake, 1997). Typically responses are characterised as a shift towards $C_{18:0}$ at the expense of $C_{16:0}$ (Banks, Clapperton, Kelly, Wilson and Crawford, 1980) due to decreased *de novo* synthesis and/or reduced mammary uptake of absorbed $C_{16:0}$ (Doreau, Chillard, Rulquin and Demeyer, 1999). Such changes are thought to arise from lowered acetate and butyrate production in the rumen associated with reductions in OM digestion and/or direct inhibition of absorbed long-chained FA on mammary *de novo* FA synthesis (Banks, Clapperton and Steele, 1983, Storry, 1981). The lack of negative effects on mammary *de novo* FA synthesis following intravenous triacylglyceride infusions suggest that the effects on rumen function are the causative factor (Grummer, 1991). Typically oil supplements decrease the proportion of saturated FA and increase both MUFA and PUFA (Table 8). Changes in milk fat unsaturated FA are characterised by small increases in the concentration of FA predominant in plant oil supplements. In all cases, feeding plant oils increase milk fat $C_{18:0}$, *cis*-9 $C_{18:1}$ and *trans* $C_{18:1}$ content due to extensive metabolism of long chain PUFA, increasing the supply of biohydrogenation intermediates and $C_{18:0}$ to the mammary gland.

Larger changes in milk FA composition can be achieved using rumen-protected lipids. Apparent transfer efficiencies of $C_{18:2}$ n-6 and $C_{18:3}$ n-3 have been increased from less than 0.05 to 0.35 and 0.42, respectively in response to formaldehyde protected lipids (Grummer, 1991). These changes are also associated with decreases in saturates and increases in MUFA and PUFA. Supplements of *cis*-9 $C_{18:1}$ acyl amide offer the promise of increasing milk fat concentrations of *cis*-9 $C_{18:1}$ up to 48 % of total FA and decrease short and medium-chain FA content (Jenkins, 1998). However, such extreme changes can be problematic due to increased risk of spontaneous oxidation and off flavours, that can to a certain extent be controlled using dietary supplements of alpha-tocopherol (Ashes, Gulati and Scott, 1997). Use of formaldehyde-treated casein encapsulation of canola/soybean oilseeds and soybean oilseed/linseed oil supplements for grazing cows increased the proportion of $C_{18:3}$ from 0.8 to 2.49 and 0.64 to 8.45 % respectively, indicating the

Table 8. Milk fatty acid responses to dietary lipid supplements

Lipid	*Inclusion*	*Mean response* [a]										*Reference*
	(g/kg DM)	$C_{14:0}$	$C_{16:0}$	$C_{18:0}$	*cis*-9 $C_{18:1}$	*trans* $C_{18:1}$	$C_{18:2}$	$C_{18:3}$	*SAT*	*MUFA*	*PUFA*	
Rapeseed oil	16	-0.03	-0.20	0.55	0.39	0.30	-0.09	0.11	-0.07	0.30	-0.04	DePeters *et al.*, 2001
Rapeseed oil	33	-0.19	-0.33	0.51	0.67	2.00	-0.04	0.60	-0.18	0.60	0.15	Loor *et al.*, 2002a
Rapeseed oil	27	-0.20	-0.25	0.36	0.35	0.66	-0.06	-0.07	-0.09	0.36	0.01	Shingfield *et al.*, unpublished
Soyabean oil	35	-0.29	-0.28	0.45	0.23	4.61	0.33	-	-0.19	0.53	0.33	Jenkins *et al.*, 1996
Soyabean oil	27	-0.21	-0.23	0.30	0.29	0.89	0.24	0.28	-0.09	0.31	0.35	Shingfield *et al.*, unpublished
Sunflower oil [b]	37	-0.32	-0.32	0.14	0.27	3.07	-0.05	-0.24	-0.22	0.53	0.12	Kalscheur *et al.*, 1997
Sunflower oil	37	-0.23	-0.26	0.15	0.11	2.79	0.07	-0.21	-0.17	0.36	0.21	Kalscheur *et al.*, 1997
Sunflower oil	50	-0.30	-0.43	0.72	0.28	3.48	0.24	-0.37	-0.15	0.65	0.40	Shingfield *et al.*, unpublished
Linseed oil	16	-0.11	-0.15	0.27	0.26	0.94	-0.14	0.17	-0.07	0.23	-0.06	Offer *et al.*, 1999
Linseed oil	27	-0.20	-0.29	0.31	0.39	0.94	-0.17	0.33	-0.11	0.39	0.26	Shingfield *et al.*, unpublished
Fish oil	16	0.04	-0.01	-0.45	-0.25	8.08	0.24	0.03	-0.09	0.24	0.29	Offer *et al.*, 1999
Fish oil	16	0.30	0.35	-0.77	-0.73	2.19	0.39	0.07	-0.05	-0.10	2.17	Shingfield *et al.*, in press
Partially hydro-genated vegetable shortening	37	-0.26	-0.18	0.02	0.16	2.72	-0.21	-0.25	-0.16	0.42	-0.05	Kalscheur *et al.*, 1997

Table 8.
Continued

Lipid	Inclusion (g/kg DM)	Mean response [a] $C_{14:0}$	$C_{16:0}$	$C_{18:0}$	*cis*-9 $C_{18:1}$	*trans* $C_{18:1}$	$C_{18:2}$	$C_{18:3}$	SAT	MUFA	PUFA	Reference
Tallow	40	-	0.06	0.04	0.22	0.19	-0.37	-0.37	-0.06	0.19	-0.36	Onetti *et al.*, 2001
White grease	40	-	0.04	0.07	0.18	0.12	-0.27	-0.23	-0.07	0.14	-0.26	Onetti *et al.*, 2001
Protected lipids												
Butylsoyamide [c]	35	-0.06	-0.05	0.04	-0.04	0.61	0.74	-	-0.04	0.01	0.74	Jenkins *et al.*, 1996
Canolamide [d]	33	-0.24	-0.33	0.76	0.74	0.93	0.04	0.40	-0.16	0.55	0.08	Loor *et al.*, 2002b
Ca-salts of rape-seed oil	40	-0.24	-0.37	0.31	0.76	-	0.10	-0.20	-0.23	0.69	0.07	Chouinard, Girard and Brisson, 1998
Ca-salts of soya-bean oil	40	-0.31	-0.37	0.35	0.73	-	0.23	-0.20	-0.23	0.63	0.19	Chouinard, Girard and Brisson, 1998
Ca-salts of lin-seed oil	40	-0.26	-0.37	0.34	0.54	-	0.36	0.40	-0.21	0.46	0.36	Chouinard, Girard and Brisson, 1998
Protected fish oil [e]	30	-	0.00	-0.36	-0.29	2.34	0.33	0.19	-0.10	0.19	0.45	Lacasse *et al.*, 2002

[a] Responses calculated as proportionate differences between treatment controls and lipid supplemented diets.
[b] High *cis*-9 $C_{18:1}$ sunflower oil.
[c] Prepared by reacting soyabean oil with butylamine
[d] Prepared by reacting rapeseed oil with ethanolamide.
[e] Encapsulated fish oil in a glutaraldehyde-treated protein matrix.

potential of this technology to effectively enhance milk n-3 PUFA content (Gulati, May, Wynn and Scott, 2002). Modifications in FA composition were also associated with changes in thermal characteristics, resulting in a proportion of liquid fat at lower temperatures, with the added benefit of improving butter spreadability (Gulati *et al.*, 2002).

Often strategies other than lipid supplementation are used to increase energy intake, including higher use of concentrate supplements and substituting grass silage for forages of higher intake potential and/or energy content. Under normal conditions, increased concentrate supplementation tends to have only minor effects on milk fat concentrations (Table 6) until the proportion of forage in the diet falls below 0.50 (Thomas and Martin, 1988) or concentrates contain relatively high levels of PUFA (Offer, Marsden, Dixon, Speake and Thacker, 1999, Offer, Marsden and Phipps, 2001b). Even though modest levels of concentrate supplements have relatively minor effects, there is evidence that the impact of concentrate feeding on milk fat content is also influenced by the composition of the basal diet. For example, Gasa, Holtenius, Sutton, Dhanoa and Napper (1991) noted that increases in concentrate supplementation from 3 to 9 kg/day caused larger decreases in milk fat content in cows fed early than late cut grass silage (5.6 and 1.1 g/kg, respectively).

It has often been thought that feeding high levels of starch are associated with milk fat depression (Keady, Mayne and Marsden, 1998, Keady *et al.*, 1999). In an attempt to establish the effects of concentrate composition on milk fat content, data based on 39 mean treatment values reported from 17 studies was subjected to meta-analysis. Replacing fibre with starch in concentrate supplements was associated with a 0.15 proportionate increase in the ratio of protein to fat (Figure 5). Even though individual experiments have shown that feeding high levels of starch are associated with milk fat depression, milk fat content of diets supplemented with starch or fibre rich concentrates in 39 comparisons was similar (mean (s.e.) 40.6 (0.64) and 40.9 (0.48) g/kg, respectively). Furthermore, in 17 cases, replacing fibre with starch in concentrate supplements decreased milk fat content. Clearly, there is little consensus between studies evaluating the effect of concentrate energy source, such that the effects of changes in concentrate composition on milk fat secretion are difficult to predict. However, in severe cases, it has been suggested that replacing cereals with soluble carbohydrates, including lactose and molasses and switching starch for digestible fibre in concentrate supplements could be used to alleviate milk fat depression on low forage diets (Sutton, 1989).

While most studies have concentrated on the use of lipid supplements, forages in the basal diet also make a significant contribution to the supply of substrates available for milk fat synthesis. In spite of the low lipid content of forages, grass silage for example, can account for proportionately 0.58 (Lock and Garnsworthy, 2002) and 0.67 (Offer *et al.*, 1999) of total FA intake. Decreases in the proportion of dietary forage are often associated with a reduction in mammary *de novo* synthesis, that are thought to reflect changes in rumen fermentation pattern, altered endocrine status causing a shift in nutrient partitioning towards adipose tissue and increases in the supply of inhibitory biohydrogenation intermediates from the rumen (Grummer, 1991, Bauman and Griinari, 2001).

Forage conservation method tends to have inconsistent effects on milk fat secretion, such that feeding hay has in some experiments increased, and in others decreased milk fat content relative to silage (Huhtanen, 1994). Manipulation of both the type and extent of silage fermentation also has variable effects on milk fat content. Use of an inoculant enzyme preparation during ensiling has reduced (Shingfield, Jaakkola and Huhtanen, 2001), marginally improved (Chamberlain, Martin, Robertson and Hunter, 1992, Mayne, 1990) or had no effect (Gordon, 1989, Keady and Murphy, 1996, Patterson, Yan, Gordon and Kilpatrick, 1998) on milk fat content.

Fresh grass contains relatively high proportions of $C_{18:3}$ (n-3) and significant amounts of $C_{18:2}$ (n-6) that are dependent on the stage of maturity (Bauchart, Vérité and Remond, 1984) and plant species (Dewhurst, Scollan, Youell, Tweed and Humphreys, 2001b). The extent to which these FA survive ensiling or drying is largely unclear, but concentrations of $C_{18:3}$ (n-3) (Aii, Takahashi, Kurihara and Kume, 1988, Hebeisen, Hoeflin, Reusch, Junker and Lauterburg, 1993, White *et al.* 2001) and conjugated linoleic acid (CLA) (Dhiman, Anand, Satter and Pariza, 1999, Jiang, Bjoerck, Fonden and Emanuelson, 1996, Kelly, Kolver, Bauman, VanAmburgh and Muller, 1998) have been consistently higher in milk produced from cows offered fresh compared with conserved forages. Exposure to solar radiation, and the duration of wilting in particular, appear to be the most important factors affecting the FA content of grass silages (Dewhurst and King, 1998) suggesting that lower concentrations of $C_{18:2}$ (n-6) and $C_{18:3}$ (n-3) in hay compared with grass silage are primarily associated with extensive oxidative losses during the drying. In spite of lower FA content, concentrations of $C_{18:2}$ (n-6) and $C_{18:3}$ (n-3) in milk are often higher for hay compared with grass silage based diets (Mansbridge and Blake, 1997).

In general, replacing grass silage with whole crop cereal silages has little effect on milk fat content, while switching to maize silage typically causes a small decrease in milk fat content, but causes an overall increase in milk fat secretion (Table 7). For grass silage based diets, milk fat content has been shown to be independent of the level N fertilizer application (Shingfield, Jaakkola and Huhtanen, 2001) or decreases in digestibility associated with advances in crop maturity (Rinne, Jaakkola, Kaustell, Heikkilä and Huhtanen, 1999b). However, the reduction in silage digestible OM content from 739 to 639 g/kg DM was associated with a curvilinear decrease in milk fat secretion.

Comparisons between the effects of forage source on the milk FA content are relatively limited. Milk fat concentrations of *cis*-9 $C_{18:1}$ and CLA are higher in pasture fed cows compared with maize silage, mountain grasses, ryegrass hay or ryegrass silage (Ferlay, Martin, Pradel, Capitan, Coulon and Chilliard, 2002). Under UK conditions, milk fat CLA and unsaturated FAs are higher during the spring and summer months as a result of higher intakes of fresh grass (Lock and Garnsworthy, 2003). Hurtaud, Delaby and Peyraud (2002a) monitored milk FA composition during the transition from a maize silage based diet to pasture. Grazing reduced short chain saturates and increased unsaturated FA content, changes that were associated with improvements in milk fat thermal characteristics, more intense colouring and reduced hardness. Comparison of the organoleptic properties of butter produced from milk from grass silage and maize silage based diets has indicated that even though maize promotes higher animal performance, butter from grass silage had better colouring and spreading characteristics (Houssin, Foret and Chenais, 2002). This may reflect the effect of these forages on milk FA composition, since concentrations of saturated FA are higher and that of $C_{18:1}$ and $C_{18:3}$ are lower in milk produced from maize silage compared with grass hay (Hurtaud, Delaby and Peyraud, 2002b).

In an attempt to predict the effect of dietary changes on milk FA composition, Hermansen (1995) used data from 35 experiments using typical lipid sources and derived relationships indicating dietary FA content was the best predictor of short chain milk FA ($<C_{12:0}$), $C_{12:0}$, $C_{14:0}$ and $C_{16:0}$ were most closely associated with their respective concentrations in the diet, whilst the best prediction of milk fat $C_{18:0}$ and $C_{18:1}$ concentrations was based on total dietary C_{18} content. Both $C_{18:2}$ (n-6) and $C_{18:3}$ (n-3) were most accurately predicted on the basis of the proportion in the diet and source of dietary lipid supplement.

Recent advances in the understanding of dietary induced milk fat depression

Production of low fat milk is an increasing and real problem for the dairy industry that can be attributed to the higher prevalence of alternative forages and use of lipid supplements to increase dietary energy content. For most production systems, development of nutritional strategies that allow marginal decreases in milk fat content are likely to improve profitability through higher levels of production for a given amount of quota. In the future, continued consumption of skimmed and semi-skimmed milk may well stimulate changes in milk pricing schemes, resulting in financial benefits for producers of low fat milk (Kennelly, 1996).

Diets that induce milk fat depression (MFD) can be broadly characterised as those containing low amounts of fibre and high starch contents or those relatively rich in PUFA. The extent of depression is more acute for diets containing low amounts of fibre and high levels of unsaturated FA (Griinari, Dwyer, McGuire, Bauman, Palmquist and Nurmela, 1998). Decreases in milk fat content typically occur within a few days after dietary changes and can be reduced by up to 50 %, with little or no change in the yield of milk or other milk constituents. In cows experiencing MFD, secretion of all FA is reduced, the extent of which is greater for short and medium chained FA (Bauman and Griinari, 2001).

Over the last 50 years a number of hypotheses have been proposed to explain dietary induced MFD. The major theories have suggested that reductions in milk fat arise from i) reductions in acetate and butyrate production in the rumen limiting mammary *de-novo* FA synthesis, ii) increased production of propionate and glucose stimulating insulin secretion causing FA to be partitioned towards adipose tissue rather than the mammary gland or iii) direct inhibition by *trans* FA produced during ruminal biohydrogenation of dietary unsaturated FA. None offer a universal explanation, but the *trans* FA hypothesis originally proposed by Davis and Brown (1970) is considered to be the most robust (Bauman and Griinari, 2001, Doreau *et al.*, 1999).

Following the observation that milk fat depression was associated with an increase in milk *trans* FA concentrations, Davis and Brown (1970) suggested that these FA directly inhibited milk fat synthesis. Numerous studies conducted across a range of diets have confirmed an inverse association between milk *trans* FA concentrations and milk fat content (Bauman and Griinari, 2001). Use of more sophisticated analytical methods (Molkentin and Precht, 1995, Wolff and Bayard, 1995) have permitted the identification of *trans*-$C_{18:1}$ isomers in milk fat with double bonds in positions Δ4-16 (Griinari *et al.*, 1998, Griinari and Shingfield, 2002, Offer *et al.*, 1999, Piperova *et al.*, 2002).

Griinari, Bauman and Jones (1995) were the first to show that the extent of MFD was related to the distribution rather than the amount of *trans*-$C_{18:1}$ secreted in milk. Subsequent studies revealed that milk fat content was inversely associated with milk fat *trans*-10 $C_{18:1}$ content (Griinari *et al.*, 1998). Newbold, Robertshaw and Morris (1998) also observed that changes in milk fat content were negatively associated with concentrations of *trans*-10 $C_{18:1}$, but unrelated to variations in *trans*-9 or *trans*-11 $C_{18:1}$. These findings confirmed earlier studies demonstrating that post-ruminal infusions of *trans*-9 $C_{18:1}$ or mixtures of *trans*-11 and 12 $C_{18:1}$ had no effect on milk fat content (Ridsig and

Schultz, 1974). More recent data has confirmed an association between milk fat *trans*-10 $C_{18:1}$ concentrations and milk fat content across a wide range of diets (Figure 7).

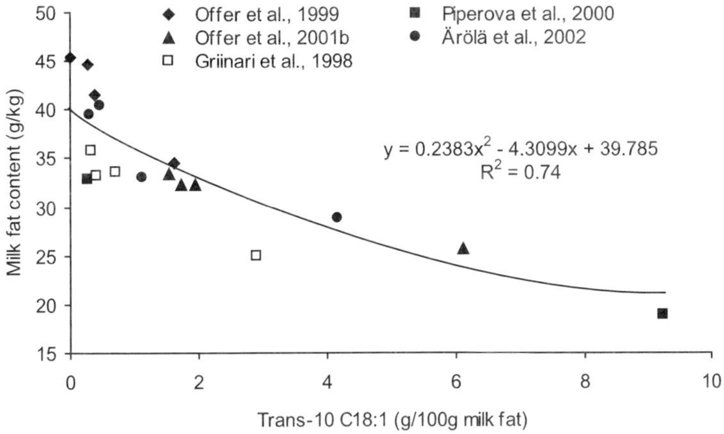

Figure 7. Relationship between milk fat content and the trans-10 $C_{18:1}$ content of milk.

In addition to the association with *trans*-10 $C_{18:1}$, a similar relationship between milk fat content and *trans*-10, *cis*-12 conjugated linoleic acid (CLA) led Griinari *et al.* (1998) to suggest that *trans*-10 $C_{18:1}$ or other related metabolites could inhibit milk fat synthesis. Loor and Herbein (1998) reported that post-ruminal infusions of a mixture of CLA isomers induced MFD, a finding subsequently confirmed by Chouinard, Corneau, Barbano, Metzger and Bauman (1999).

More recently, post-ruminal infusions of *trans*-10, *cis*-12 $C_{18:2}$ have been shown to induce a 40 % reduction in milk fat content, proportionately 0.78 of which was due to decreased *de novo* FA synthesis, while infusions of *cis*-9, *trans*-11 $C_{18:2}$ have no effect (Baumgard, Corl, Dwyer, Sæbø and Bauman, 2000, Figure 8). Further studies have shown that post-ruminal infusions of 2.5 or 14 g/day of *trans*-10, *cis*-12 isomer result in a proportionate reductions in milk fat yield of 0.17 (Peterson, Baumgard and Bauman, 2002) and 0.50 (Baumgard, Sangster and Bauman, 2001), respectively. Examining data reported in the literature provides compelling evidence of inhibitory effects of *trans*-10, *cis*-12 $C_{18:2}$ on milk fat content and yield (Figure 9). Perhaps the most interesting aspect of these studies is that the responses to *trans*-10, *cis*-12 $C_{18:2}$ infusions are consistent with changes that occur during dietary induced MFD (Bauman and Griinari, 2001). The increase in milk *trans*-10 $C_{18:1}$ and *trans*-10, *cis*-12 $C_{18:2}$ content during MFD has promoted the suggestion that CLA isomers containing a *trans*-10 double bond are responsible (Baumgard *et al.*, 2000). However, preliminary investigations have indicated that *cis*-8, *trans*-10 $C_{18:2}$ does not exert these effects (Perfield, Sæbø and Bauman, 2003) and there is no direct evidence that *trans*-10 $C_{18:1}$ inhibits milk fat synthesis.

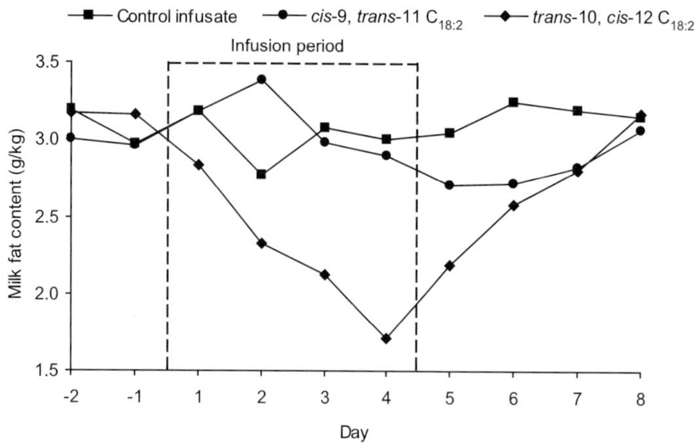

Figure 8. Effect of abomasal infusions (10g/day) of control infusate, cis-9, trans-11 $C_{18:2}$, and trans-10, cis 12 $C_{18:2}$ on milk fat content (data derived from Baumgard *et al.*, 2000)

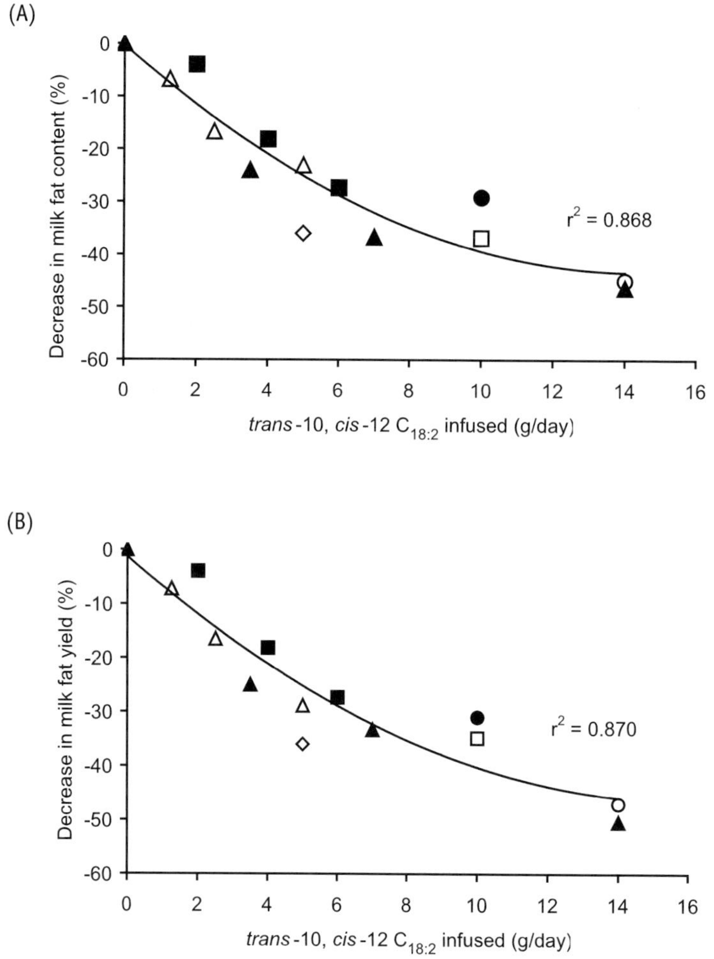

Figure 9. Effect of *trans*-10, *cis*-12 $C_{18:2}$ on the percentage decrease in (A) milk fat content and (B) yield (B) in lactating dairy cows. Data from ▲ Baumgard, Sangster and Bauman (2001); ● Baumgard *et al.* (2000a); □ Baumgard *et al.* (2000b); ○ Matitashvili, Baumgard and Bauman (2001); △ Peterson, Baumgard and Bauman (2002) and ◇ Loor *et al.* (2002a) based on abomasal infusions, and ■ Viswanadha, Hanson, Giesy and McGuire (2000) based on intravenous administration.

The underlying mechanism for the decreases in milk fat content appear to be related to an inhibition in a number of key enzymes involved in milk fat synthesis. Feeding diets that cause MFD also induce reductions in mammary acetyl-CoA carboxylase and fatty acid synthase activity (Piperova, Teter, Bruckental, Sampugna, Mills, Yurawecz, Fritsche, Ku and Erdman, 2000), whilst post-ruminal infusions of *trans*-10, *cis*-12 $C_{18:2}$ have been shown to decrease mRNA expression for acetyl-CoA carboxylase, fatty acid synthase, Δ^9-desaturase, lipoprotein lipase, fatty acid binding protein, glycerol phosphate acyltransferase and acylglycerol phosphate acyltransferase (Baumgard, Matitashvili, Corl, Dwyer, and Bauman, 2002).

In light of the proposal of Davis and Brown (1970) that *trans*-$C_{18:1}$ FA inhibit milk fat synthesis, Bauman and Griinari (2001) reported the necessity for updating this hypothesis to account for the most recent findings. A 'biohydrogenation theory' was proposed on the basis that dietary conditions resulting in MFD alter rumen biohydrogenation pathways, and hence encourage the formation of unique biohydrogenation intermediates that inhibit milk fat synthesis in the mammary gland (Bauman and Griinari, 2001).

Even though infusion studies have demonstrated the potent effects of *trans*-10, *cis*-12 $C_{18:2}$ on milk fat synthesis, MFD can occur in the absence of increases in the concentration of this isomer in milk fat. For example, fish oil supplementation of grass silage based diets rich in $C_{18:3}$ (n-3) generally induce MFD but have only minor effects on milk fat *trans*-10, *cis*-12 $C_{18:2}$ concentrations (Ärölä, Shingfield, Vanhatalo, Toivonen, Huhtanen and Griinari, 2002, Offer *et al.*, 1999). In such cases, Bauman and Griinari (2001) highlighted the possibility that other FA such as conjugated $C_{18:3}$ FA may be responsible.

Changing milk composition for improved human health

The important role of milk as a versatile source of nutrients is well established. In addition to traditional attributes there is a growing body of evidence that the consumption of milk and dairy products may confer additional benefits with respect to the diseases of ageing, including cancer, atherosclerosis and other degenerative disorders (Parodi, 1994). Specific proteins, peptides and FA are thought to be the active components, while the production of fermented milk products have also been shown to have the potential to elicit beneficial effects (Heller, 2001, Sanders, 1998).

Cardiovascular disease

Cardiovascular disease (CVD), principally coronary heart disease and stroke and cancer are the principal causes of death in the UK. The major determinants of CVD risk are smoking, blood pressure levels, blood cholesterol concentrations and physical inactivity (Wiseman, 1997). Over consumption of energy coupled with a relatively inactive lifestyle has led to a dramatic increase in the incidence of obesity that is also associated with CVD risk, partly due to elevated blood pressure and plasma cholesterol levels. On the basis of epidemiological and intervention studies in human subjects it has been generally accepted that saturated FA increase blood cholesterol concentrations in a predictable and dose dependent manner (Hegsted, McGandy and Myers, 1965, Keys, Anderson and Grande, 1965). It is perhaps not surprising that National nutritional guidelines with a view to reducing the incidence of coronary health disease advocate a reduction in the intake of total fat and saturated FA (COMA, 1984, COMA, 1994). Publication of the original COMA report has been the foundation of public health policy in the UK. Unfortunately, dissemination of this report has created a general perception that animal fats are synonymous with saturated FA and hence increased CVD risk, whilst the underlying hypothesis and conclusions of the report have been criticised for failing to establish a causative link between the amount and type of dietary fat relative to CVD risk (Blaxter and Webster, 1991, Gurr, 1999). Furthermore, when considering dietary effects on human health related outcomes it is important to recognise that levels of LDL cholesterol are positively associated with CVD risk, but HDL cholesterol exert a protective effect (Maniapane and Salter, 1999, Maijala, 2000).

Currently total fat intake of human subjects in Western Europe accounts for about 40 % of total daily energy intake, equivalent to 130 g/day (Demeyer and Doreau, 1999). Milk and dairy products are a major source of fats in the human diet and thought to contribute to 30 and 40 % of total and saturated fat intake in the UK, respectively (Mansbridge and Blake, 1997). Milk fat typically contains proportionately between 0.70 and 0.75 saturated fatty acids (SFA), 0.25 and 0.20 MUFA and relatively minor amounts of PUFA (Table 9).

Even though $C_{18:0}$ (Bonanome and Grundy, 1988) and the short-chained SFA ($C_{4:0}$ - $C_{10:0}$) are essentially neutral (Blaxter and Webster, 1991), $C_{12:0}$, $C_{14:0}$ and $C_{16:0}$ that account for the majority of SFA in milk fat have been implicated for increases in total and LDL cholesterol concentrations (Williams, 2000). Milk fat is the predominant source of $C_{4:0}$ - $C_{10:0}$, $C_{12:0}$ and $C_{14:0}$ in the diet (Gunstone, Harwood and Padley, 1994) and as such consumption of milk and dairy products would be expected to have adverse effects on plasma cholesterol levels. However, the evidence from studies in adolescents (Samuelson, Bratteby, Mohsen and Vessby, 2001) and elderly men (Smedman, Gustafsson, Berglund and Vessby, 1999) suggests that consumption of milk and dairy products do not necessarily exert the expected detrimental effects on blood lipids, and may, in fact, elicit beneficial effects (Buonopane, Kilara, Smith and

Table 9. Typical fatty acid composition of bovine milk fat

Fatty acid	g/100g total fatty acids
$C_{4:0}$	4.58
$C_{6:0}$	2.23
$C_{8:0}$	1.11
$C_{10:0}$	2.22
$C_{12:0}$	2.40
$C_{14:0}$	10.2
$C_{14:1}$ (n-5)	0.56
$C_{16:0}$	24.7
$C_{16:1}$ (n-7)	1.29
$C_{18:0}$	19.54
$C_{18:1}$ *cis*-9	18.11
$C_{18:1}$ *cis*-11	0.59
$C_{18:1}$ *cis*-12	0.18
$C_{18:1}$ *cis* total	19.0
$C_{18:1}$ *trans*-6,-7 and-8	0.26
$C_{18:1}$ *trans*-9	0.26
$C_{18:1}$ *trans*-10	0.21
$C_{18:1}$ *trans*-11	1.80
$C_{18:1}$ *trans*-12	0.34
$C_{18:1}$ *trans*-13 and -14	0.63
$C_{18:1}$ *trans*-15	0.50
$C_{18:1}$ *trans*-16	0.46
$C_{18:1}$ *trans* total	4.51
$C_{18:2}$ (n-6)	0.90
$C_{18:2}$ *trans*-11, *cis*-15	0.19
$C_{18:2}$ *trans*, *trans*	0.10
$C_{18:2}$ total‡	1.41
Cis-9, *trans*-11 $C_{18:2}$	0.39
trans-7, *cis*-9 $C_{18:2}$	0.03
trans-11, *cis*-13 $C_{18:2}$	0.04
CLA total	0.56
$C_{18:3}$ (n-3)	0.42
$C_{20:0}$	0.90
$C_{20:1}$ (n-9)	0.23
$C_{20:5}$ (n-3)	0.05
$C_{24:0}$	0.04
Summary	
Total = C14	23.2
Total saturates	71.0
Total monounsaturates	26.0
Total polyunsaturates	2.52
Total (n-3) polyunsaturates	0.51

‡sum of $C_{18:2}$ excluding isomers of CLA.
Adapted from Shingfield *et al*. (2003a)

McCarthy, 1992). Furthermore, a recent prospective study examining the relationship between milk and coronary heart disease concluded that there was no association between the consumption of whole fat milk and death from CVD (Ness, Smith and Hart, 2001).

Following the findings that replacement of saturated fat with MUFA has a protective effect against CVD (Keys, Menotti, Karvonen, Aravanis, Blackburn, Buzina, Djordjevic, Dontas, Fidanza and Keys, 1986) numerous trials have confirmed the hypocholesterolaemic effect of isoenergetic replacement of saturated FA with MUFA in human diets (Williams, 2000). Consumption of MUFA enriched dairy products from milk produced from cows fed fomaldehyde-casein treated rapeseed and soyabean oil has been shown to induce significant 0.043 and 0.053 proportionate reductions in total and LDL cholesterol concentrations (Noakes, Nestel and Clifton, 1996). Poppitt, Keogh, Mulvey, McArdle, MacGibbon and Cooper (2002) reported similar responses of 0.079 and 0.095 in subjects offered modified butter. In contrast, an intervention study comparing typical butter with that enriched with MUFA produced from cows fed supplements of crushed rapeseeds had no influence on these blood lipid fractions, but increased plasma triacylglyceride levels, an effect thought to be related to increases in milk fat trans $C_{18:1}$ content (Tholstrup, Sandstrom, Hermansen and Holmer, 1998). Whilst there is some discrepancy between these studies that can be related to differences in methodology, the general conclusion to be drawn is that manipulation of milk FA composition towards longer chain SFA, MUFA and PUFA at the expense of short and medium chain SFA has the potential to favourably alter blood lipids (Table 10). Furthermore, the decreases in LDL attained using dairy products modified using rumen-protected lipids are similar to those when whole milk has been replaced in the diet with skimmed milk (Buonopane *et al.*, 1992, Steinmetz, Childs, Stimson, Kushi, McGovern, Potter and Yamanaka, 1994).

Attempts to manipulate milk FA composition towards long chain saturated FA and MUFA using oilseeds or free oil result in an unavoidable elevation in milk fat trans $C_{18:1}$ content (Jensen, 2002) due to increased ruminal synthesis. Trans FA raise plasma total and LDL cholesterol concentrations (Mensink and Katan, 1990), but in contrast to saturated FA, also lower HDL cholesterol when substituted for cis unsaturated FAs (Williams, 2000, Zock and Katan, 1997). The implication is that high consumption of trans FA is associated with increased CVD risk. Further examination of LDL cholesterol responses (Willett, Stampfer, Manson, Colditz, Speizer, Rosner, Sampson and Hennekens, 1993) suggest that *trans*-9 and *trans*-10 $C_{18:1}$, prevalent in partially hydrogenated vegetable oils are more potent than *trans*-11 $C_{18:1}$ the predominant isomer in milk fat (Griinari and Shingfield, 2002). Whilst the distribution and concentration of trans isomers is markedly different between hydrogenated plant oils and milk fat (Table 11) the impact of increases in trans $C_{18:1}$ and $C_{18:2}$ FA during attempts to manipulate milk FA composition on human plasma lipid profiles merits further investigation.

Table 10. Effect of consumption of modified dairy products on plasma lipids in human subjects.

Study Composition (g/100g total fatty acids)	*Noakes et al. 1996* Control	Modified	*Tholstrup et al. 1998* Control	Modified	*Poppitt et al. 2002* Control	Modified
$C_{12:0}$	3.3	2.3	4.1	2.9	3.8	2.7
$C_{14:0}$	10.0	6.7	12.1	10.7	12.0	8.3
$C_{16:0}$	25.9	15.5	36.8	21.1	31.5	18.8
$C_{18:0}$	11.7	14.3	7.2	10.9	10.1	13.4
$C_{18:1}$ *cis*-9	22.8	35.3	15.3	25.0	14.3	25.3
$C_{18:1}$ *trans*	NR	NR	1.1	6.4	4.3	4.7
$C_{18:1}$ total	NR	NR	17.0	32.8	18.6	30.0
$C_{18:2}$ (n-6)	1.5	6.9	1.6	1.9	1.2	7.2
$C_{18:3}$ (n-3)	0.7	2.2	0.4	0.5	0.8	2.3
Plasma concentrations (mmol/l)						
Total cholesterol	6.50	6.22***	4.31	4.24	4.31	4.22*
LDL cholesterol	4.49	4.25***	2.89	2.83	2.85	2.70**
HDL cholesterol	1.30	1.28	1.20	1.13	1.16	1.19
Triglycerides	1.57	1.54	0.85	0.99	0.69	0.74

NR: not reported
*, ** and * refer to significant differences between the control and modified fat treatment at $P < 0.05$, < 0.01 and < 0.001, respectively.
*** $P < 0.001$

Intakes of saturated fat in the United Kingdom currently account for 15 % of total energy (Department of the Environment, 2001) that exceed recommended levels of 10 % (COMA, 1994), and therefore replacement of saturated with cis containing MUFA could be used as part of the public health policy to reduce CVD risk (Sanderson, Gill, Packard, Sanders, Vessby and Williams, 2002). In essence, modification of milk FA composition could be used as an integral component of an overall strategy to improve the health of the nation.

Cancer

It has been suggested that about 35 % of all cancer deaths can be directly attributed to diet (Doll, 1992). A number of long-term

Table 11. Concentration of trans $C_{18:1}$ fatty acids in edible fats (g/100g total fatty acids)

Positional isomer	Margarines			Shortenings			Bovine milk fat		
	Min	*Max*	*Mean*	*Min*	*Max*	*Mean*	*Min*	*Max*	*Mean*
$C_{18:1}$ *trans*-4	0.00	0.11	0.03	0.00	0.12	0.03	0.02	0.08	0.05
$C_{18:1}$ *trans*-5	0.00	0.16	0.06	0.00	0.29	0.08	0.00	0.11	0.05
$C_{18:1}$ *trans*-6,-7 and-8	0.02	3.90	1.63	0.00	5.32	1.54	0.07	0.27	0.16
$C_{18:1}$ *trans*-9	0.05	4.84	2.04	0.01	6.52	2.28	0.16	0.30	0.23
$C_{18:1}$ *trans*-10	0.04	5.30	1.93	0.01	6.74	1.98	0.03	0.30	0.17
$C_{18:1}$ *trans*-11	0.03	4.50	1.38	0.01	5.19	1.45	0.35	4.43	1.72
$C_{18:1}$ *trans*-12	0.02	4.08	1.12	0.00	4.06	1.19	0.10	0.31	0.21
$C_{18:1}$ *trans*-13 and -14	0.01	3.56	0.92	0.00	3.25	0.97	0.00	0.85	0.49
$C_{18:1}$ *trans*-15	0.00	0.45	0.13	0.00	0.67	0.18	0.04	0.48	0.28
$C_{18:1}$ *trans*-16	0.00	0.53	0.09	0.00	0.35	0.10	0.11	0.52	0.33
$C_{18:1}$ total *trans*	0.17	25.90	9.32	0.04	32.51	9.79	0.88	7.65	3.69

Adapted from Precht and Molkentin (1995).

epidemiological studies have examined the impact of milk and dairy product consumption on the incidence of various cancers. Patients suffering from cancer of the bladder were found to have a far lower intakes or complete abstention from milk products compared with a healthy control group (Mettlin and Graham, 1979), while the outcome of a twenty-five year follow-up study established an inverse relationship between the intake of dairy products and breast cancer risk (Knekt, Jarvinen, Seppanen, Pukkala and Aromaa, 1996).

Protective effects appear to be related with several compounds, some of which are specific to milk. Butyric acid ($C_{4:0}$) exhibits anti-neoplastic properties and inhibits the growth of a number of cancer cell lines, including those of the breast and colon (Parodi, 1997). Ether lipids present in milk also possess anti-proliferative properties at very low concentrations (Parodi, 1997) that are thought to inhibit the growth, anti-metastatic activity and induction of differentiation and apoptosis of cancer cells (Molkentin, 2000).

Early work demonstrated that extracts of fried ground beef contained compounds that inhibited mutagenesis (Pariza, Ashoor, Chu and Lund, 1979). Further work identified that these effects were due to a mixture of conjugated cis-9, trans-11, trans-9, trans-11, trans-10, cis-12 and trans-10, trans-12 $C_{18:2}$ FA (Ha, Grimm and Pariza, 1987). Thereafter, considerable evidence has been accrued to support the beneficial effects of CLA mixtures with respect to inhibition of human cancer cell lines and suppression of chemically induced tumour development (Kritchevsky, 2000, Parodi, 1999). Anti-carcinogenic properties are attributable to the cis-9, trans-11 isomer (Ip et al., 1999), which also happens to be the predominant CLA isomer in milk fat (Chin, Liu, Storkson, Ha and Pariza, 1992).

Conclusions and future perspectives

Milk is a valuable source of nutrients providing energy, high quality protein, and essential minerals and vitamins to the human diet, but the consumption of milk and dairy products has fallen considerably over the past 30 years. Nutrition can be used as an effective strategy to effect considerable changes in milk composition. The impact of manipulating nutrient supply on milk protein content is relatively minor compared with genetic potential. Milk protein concentrations can be increased when grass silage is replaced with maize silage or through more intense concentrate feeding, while lipid supplements have a negative effect. Responses to AA are generally realised as higher milk protein yields than increases in milk protein content. Nutrition has a much greater impact on milk fat content. Milk fat content increases when the supply of absorbed AA is not balanced with respect to requirements for milk protein synthesis or through dietary inclusion of rumen protected tallow. In most cases, lipids decrease milk fat content, the extent of which is dependent on level of inclusion, degree of unsaturation and composition of the basal diet. A number of theories have been proposed to explain the underlying causes of milk fat depression. The most scientifically convincing is related to increased ruminal production of biohydrogenation intermediates that elicit inhibitory effects on mammary FA synthesis. Clearly, *trans*-10, *cis*-12 is a potent inhibitor of milk fat synthesis, but changes in the formation of this isomer in the rumen, may not exclusively account for dietary induced changes in milk fat content. Lipid supplements can be used as an effective strategy for manipulating milk FA composition. Supplements of long-chained FA decrease FA synthesised *de novo*, and increase the proportion of unsaturated FA in milk fat. The magnitude of response is related to the form, degree of unsaturation and extent of ruminal biohydrogenation of lipid supplements and the composition of the basal diet. In all cases, attempts to enhance milk fat concentrations of monounsaturated, conjugated linoleic acid and polyunsaturated fatty acids, and reduce saturates result in an unavoidable increase in *trans* FA content, the impact on human health related outcomes remains uncertain. Development of niche markets for milk enriched with specific FA of known efficacy is dependent on further clarification of these effects. Milk in its present form contains a number of components that appear to have positive effects with respect to chronic diseases such as CVD and cancer. Epidemiological evidence is not consistent with the view that consumption of milk and dairy products is necessarily detrimental to human health. Milk fat contains over 400 different fatty acids, and it would not be surprising if one or more of these as yet uninvestigated compounds also possess bioactive properties. The prospect for the dairy industry to respond to these exciting opportunities is dependent on a multidisciplinary consensus on the milk fatty acid profiles necessary for improved human health. Increasing the levels of such compounds in milk and dairy products, coupled with a re-emphasis of the well documented positive attributes, would undoubtedly improve the perception of milk and dairy products by consumers and thereby enhance the profitability of dairy enterprises, but may also confer significant benefits to the health of the nation.

References

Agricultural Research Council. 1984. The Nutrient Requirements of Ruminant Livestock. Supplement 1. Commonwealth Agricultural Bureaux, Farningham Royal, Slough, UK.

Ahnadi, C.E., Beswick, N., Delbecchi, L., Kennelly J.J. and Lacasse P. (2002) Addition of fish oil to diets for dairy cows. II. Effects on milk fat and gene expression of mammary lipogenic enzymes.

Journal of Dairy Research, **69**: 521-531.
Aii T., Takahashi, S., Kurihara, M. and Kume, S. (1988) The effects of Italian ryegrass hay, haylage and fresh Italian ryegrass on the fatty acid composition of cows' milk. *Japanese Journal of Zootechnical Science*, **59**: 718-724.
Ärölä, A., Shingfield, K. J., Vanhatalo, A., Toivonen, V., Huhtanen, P. and Griinari, J. M. (2002) Biohydrogenation shift and milk fat depression in lactating dairy cows fed increasing levels of fish oil. *Journal of Dairy Science*, **85 (Suppl. 1)**: 143.
Ashes, J.R., Gulati, S.K. and Scott, T.W. (1997) Potential to alter the content and composition of milk fat through nutrition. *Journal of Dairy Science*, **80**: 2204-2212.
Aston, K., Thomas, C., Daley, S.R. and Sutton J.D. (1994) Milk production from grass-silage diets - Effects of the composition of supplementary concentrates. *Animal Production*, **59**: 335-344.
Auldist, M.J., Walsh, B.J. and Thomson, N.A. (1998) Seasonal and lactational influences on bovine milk composition in New Zealand. *Journal of Dairy Research*, **65**: 401-411.
Banks, W., Clapperton, J.L., Kelly, M.E., Wilson, A.G. and Crawford R.J.M. (1980) The yield, fatty acid composition and physical properties of milk fat obtained by feeding soya oil to dairy cows. *Journal of the Science of Food and Agriculture*, **31**: 368-374.
Banks, W., Clapperton, J.L. and Steele W. (1983) Dietary manipulation of the content and fatty acid composition of milk fat. *Proceedings of the Nutrition Society*, **42**: 399-406.
Bauchart, D., Legay-Carmier, F., Doreau, M. and Gaillard, B. (1990) Lipid metabolism of liquid-associated and solid-adherent bacteria in rumen contents of dairy cows offered lipid-supplemented diets. *British Journal of Nutrition*, **63**: 563-578.
Bauchart, D., Vérité, R. and Remond, B. (1984) Long-chain fatty acid digestion in lactating cows fed fresh grass from spring to autumn. *Candian Journal of Animal Science*, **64 (Suppl. 1)**: 330-331.
Bauman, D. E. (2000) Regulation of nutrient partitioning during lactation: homeostasis and homeorhesis revisited. Pages 311-327 in *Ruminant Physiology: Digestion, Metabolism and Growth and Reproduction*. P. J. Cronje, ed. CAB Publishing, New York, USA.
Bauman, D.E. and Davis C.L. (1974) Biosynthesis of milk fat. Pages 31-75 in *Lactation: a comprehensive treatise*. B.L. Larson and V.R. Smith, eds. Academic Press, London, UK.
Bauman, D.E. and Griinari, J. M. (2001) Regulation and nutritional manipulation of milk fat: low-fat milk syndrome. *Livestock Production Science*, **70**: 15-29.
Baumgard, L.H., Corl, B.A., Dwyer, D.A., Sæbø, A. and Bauman, D.E. (2000) Identification of the conjugated linoleic acid isomer that inhibits milk fat synthesis. *American Journal of Physiology*, **278**: R179-R184.
Baumgard, L.H., Matitashvili, E. Corl, B.A., Dwyer, D.A. and Bauman,

D.E. (2002) *trans*-10, *cis*-12 CLA decreases lipogenic rates and expression of genes involved in milk lipid synthesis in dairy cows. *Journal of Dairy Science*, **85**: 2155-2163.

Baumgard, L.H., J.K. Sangster, and D.E. Bauman. (2001) Milk fat synthesis in dairy cows is progressively reduced by increasing amounts of *trans*-10, *cis*-12 conjugated linoleic acid. *Journal of Nutrition*, **131**: 1764-1769.

Beaulieu, A.D. and Palmquist, D.L. (1995) Differential effects of high fat diets on fatty acid composition in milk of Jersey and Holstein cows. *Journal of Dairy Science*, **78**: 1336-1344.

Beever, D.E. (1993) Rumen function. Pages 186-215 in *Quantitative aspects of ruminant digestion and metabolism*. J.M. Forbes and J.France, eds. CAB International, Wallingford, UK.

Bequette, B.J., Backwell, F.R.C. and Crompton, L.A. (1998) Current concepts of amino acid and protein metabolism in the mammary gland of the lactating ruminant. *Journal of Dairy Science*, **81**: 2540-2559.

Bickerstaffe, R., Annison, E.F. and Linzell, J.L. (1974) The metabolism of glucose, acetate, lipids and amino acids in lactating dairy cows. *Journal of Agricultural Science, Cambridge*, **82**: 85-90.

Black, A.L., Anand, R.S., Bruss, M.L., Brown, C.D. and Nakagiri, JA. (1990) Partitioning of amino acids in lactating cows: Oxidation to carbon dioxide. *Journal of Nutrition*, **120**: 700-710.

Blaxter, K.L. and Webster, A.J.F. (1991) Animal production and food: problems and paranoia. *Animal Production*, **53**: 261-269.

Bonanome, A. and Grundy, S. M. (1988) Effect of dietary stearic-acid on plasma-cholesterol and lipoprotein levels. *New England Journal of Medicine*, **318**: 1244-1248.

Buonopane, G.J., Kilara, A., Smith, J.S. and McCarthy, R.D. (1992) Effect of skimmed milk supplementation on blood cholesterol concentration, blood pressure and triglycerides in a free-living human population. *Journal of the American College of Nutrition*, **11**: 56-67.

Brockman, R. P. (1993) Glucose and short-chain fatty acid metabolism. Pages 249-265 in *Quantitative aspects of ruminant digestion and metabolism*. J. M. Forbes and J. France, eds. CAB International, Wallingford, UK.

Broderick, G.A. and Merchen, N.R. (1992) Markers for quantifying microbial protein synthesis in the rumen. *Journal of Dairy Science*, **75**: 2618-2632.

Broderick, G.A., Mertens, D.R. and Simons, R. (2002) Efficacy of carbohydrate sources for milk production by cows fed diets based on alfalfa silage. *Journal of Dairy Science*, **85**: 1767-1776.

Cant, J. P., Berthiaume, R., Lapierre, H., Luimes, P.H., McBride, B.W. and Pacheco, D. (2002) Responses of the bovine mammary glands to absorptive supply of single amino acids. Pages 27-43 in Canadian Society of Animal Science Symposium "*Amino acids:*

milk, meat and more!"

Castle, M.E., Gill, M.S. and Watson, J.N. (1981) Silage and milk-production - a comparison between barley and dried sugar-beet pulp as silage supplements. *Grass and Forage Science*, **36**: 319-324.

Chamberlain, D.G. and Choung J.J. (1995) The importance of rate of ruminal fermentation of energy sources in diets for dairy cows. Pages 3-27 in *Recent Advances in Animal Nutrition 1985*. P. C. Garnsworthy and D.J.A. Cole, eds. Nottingham University Press, Nottingham, UK.

Chamberlain, D.G., Martin, P.A. and Robertson, S. (1989) Optimising compund feed use in dairy cows with high intakes of silage. Pages 175-193 in *Recent Advances in Animal Nutrition 1989*. W. Haresign and D.J.A. Cole, eds. Butterworth, London.

Chamberlain, D.G., Martin, P.A., Robertson, S. and Hunter, E.A. (1992) Effects of the type of additive and the type of supplement on the utilization of grass silage for milk production in dairy cows. *Grass and Forage Science*, **47**: 391-399.

Chamberlain, D.G., Thomas, P.C., Wilson, W.D., Kassem, M.E. and Robertson, S. (1984) The influence of the type of carbohydrate in the supplementary concentrate on the utilisation of silage diets for milk production. Proceedings of the Seventh Silage Conference, Queens University, Belfast: 37-38.

Chilliard, Y. (1993) Dietary fat and adipose tissue metabolism in ruminants, pigs, and rodents: A review. *Journal of Dairy Science*, **76**: 3897-3931.

Chilliard, Y. and Doreau, M. (1997) Influence of supplementary fish oil and rumen-protected methionine on milk yield and composition in dairy cows. *Journal of Dairy Research*, **64**: 173-179.

Chilliard, Y., Ferlay, A. and Doreau, M. (2001) Effect of different types of forages, animal fat or marine oils in cow's diet on milk fat secretion and composition, especially conjugated linoleic acid (CLA) and polyunsaturated fatty acids. *Livestock Production Science*, **70**: 31-48.

Chillard, Y., Ferlay, A., Mansbridge, R.M. and Doreau M. (2000) Ruminant milk fat plasticity: nutritional control of saturated, polyunsaturated, trans and conjugated fatty acids. *Annales de Zootechnie*, **49**: 181-205.

Chin, S.F., Liu, W., Storkson, J.M., Ha, Y.L. and Pariza, M.W. (1992) Dietary sources of dienoic isomers of linoleic acid, a newly recognised class of anticarcinogins. *Journal of Food Composition and Analysis*, **5**: 185-197.

Chouinard, P.Y., Girard, V. and Brisson G.J. (1998) Fatty acid profile and physical properties of milk fat from cows fed calcium salts of fatty acids with varying unsaturation. *Journal of Dairy Science*, **81**: 471-481.

Chouinard, P.Y., Corneau, L., Barbano, D.M., Metzger, L.E. and Bauman

D.E. (1999) Conjugated linoleic acids alter milk fatty acid composition and inhibit milk fat secretion in dairy cows. *Journal of Nutrition*, **129**: 1579-1584.

Choung, J.J. and Chamberlain, D.G. (1992) Protein nutrition of dairy cows receiving grass silage based diets. Effects on silage intake and milk production of postruminal supplements of casein or soya-bean-protein isolate and the effects of intravenous infusions of a mixture of methionine, phenylalanine and tryptophan. *Journal of the Science of Food and Agriculture*, **58**: 380-386.

Christie, W.W. (1981) The composition, structure and function of lipids in the tissues of ruminant animals. Pages 95-191 in *Lipid metabolism in ruminant animals*. W. W. Christie, ed. Pergamon Press Ltd., Oxford, UK.

Christie, W.W. (1995) Composition and structure of milk lipids. Pages 1-36 in *Advanced Dairy Chemistry Volume 2: Lipids*. P. F. Fox, ed. Chapman and Hall, London, UK.

Clark, J.H. (1975) Lactational responses to postruminal administration of proteins and amino acids. *Journal of Dairy Science*, **58**: 1178-1197.

Clark, J.H., Klusmeyer, T.H. and Cameron, M.R. (1992) Microbial protein synthesis and flows of nitrogen fractions and amino acid nutrition in dairy cattle. *Journal of Dairy Science*, **75**: 2304-2323.

Committee on Medical Aspects of Food Policy. (1984) Diet and cardiovascular disease. Department of Health and Social Security report on health and social subjects No. 28. HMSO, London, UK.

Committee on Medical Aspects of Food Policy. (1994) Nutritional aspects of cardiovascular disease. Department of Health and Social Security report on health and social subjects No. 46. HMSO, London, UK.

Corl, B.A., Baumgard, L.H., Griinari, J.M. Delmonte, P., Morehouse, K.M., Yuraweczc, M.P. and Bauman D.E. (2002) *Trans-7, cis-9* CLA is synthesized endogenously by delta 9-desaturase in dairy cows. *Lipids*, **37**:681-688.

Coulon, J.B., Hurtaud, C., Remond, B. and Vérité, R. (1998) Factors contributing to variation in the proportion of casein in cows' milk true protein: a review of recent INRA experiments. *Journal of Dairy Research*, **65**: 375-387.

Coulon, J.B. and Remond, B. (1991) Variations in milk output and milk protein-content in response to the level of energy supply to the dairy-cow - a review. *Livestock Production Science*, **29**: 31-47.

Danfær, A., Tetens, V. and Agergaard, N. (1995) Review and an experimental-study on the physiological and quantitative aspects of gluconeogenesis in lactating ruminants. *Comparative Biochemistry and Physiology B-Biochemistry and Molecular Biology*, **111**: 201-210.

Davis, C.L. and Brown, R.E. (1970) Low-fat milk syndrome. Pages 545-

565 in *Physiology of digestion and metabolism in the ruminant*. A. T. Phillipson, ed. Oriel Press, Newcastle upon Tyne, UK.

Delbecchi, L., Ahnadi, C.E., Kennelly, J.J. and Lacasse, P. (2001) Milk fatty acid composition and mammary lipid metabolism in Holstein cows fed protected or unprotected canola seeds. *Journal of Dairy Science*, **84**: 1375-1381.

Demeyer, D. and Doreau, M. (1999) Targets and procedures for altering ruminant meat and milk lipids. *Proceedings of the Nutrition Society*, **58**: 593-607.

Department of the Environment, Food and Rural Affairs. (2001) The National Food Survey. HMSO, London. Available at: www.defra.gov.uk/esg/m_natstats.htm

DePeters, E. J. and J. P. Cant. (1992) Nutritional factors influencing the nitrogen composition of bovine milk: a review. *Journal of Dairy Science*, **75**: 2043-2070.

DePeters, E.J., German, J.B., Taylor, S.J., Essex, S.T. and Perez-Monti, H. (2001) Fatty acid and triglyceride composition of milk fat from lactating Holstein cows in response to supplemental canola oil. *Journal of Dairy Science*, **84**: 929-936.

Dewhurst, R. J., Aston, K., Fisher, W.J., Evans, R.T., Dhanoa, M.S. and McAllan, A.B. (1999) Comparison of energy and protein sources offered at low levels in grass-silage-based diets for dairy cows. *Animal Science*, **68**: 789-799.

Dewhurst, R.J., Davies, D.R., and Merry, R.J. (2000) Microbial protein supply from the rumen. *Animal Feed Science and Technology*, **85**: 1-21.

Dewhurst, R.J., Hepper, D. and Webster, A.J.F. (1995) Comparison of in sacco and in vitro techniques for estimating the rate and extent of rumen fermentation of a range of dietary ingredients. *Animal Feed Science and Technology*, **51**: 211-229.

Dewhurst, R.J. and King, P.J. (1998) Effects of extended wilting, shading and chemical additives on the fatty acids in laboratory grass silages. *Grass and Forage Science*, **53**: 219-224.

Dewhurst R.J., Scollan, N.D., Youell, S.J., Tweed, J.K.S. and Humphreys, M.O. (2001b) Influence of species, cutting date and cutting interval on the fatty acid composition of grasses. *Grass and Forage Science*, **56**: 68-74.

Dewhurst, R. J., Wadhwa, D., Borgida, L.P. and Fisher, W.J. (2001a) Rumen acid production from dairy feeds. 1. Effects on feed intake and milk production of dairy cows offered grass or corn silages. *Journal of Dairy Science*, **84**: 2721-2729.

Dhiman, T.R., Anand, G.R., Satter, L.D. and Pariza, M.W. (1999) Conjugated linoleic acid content of milk from cows fed different diets. *Journal of Dairy Science*, **82**: 2146-2156.

Doll, R. (1992) The lessons of life: keynote address to the Nutrition and Cancer Conference. *Cancer Research*. **52**: S2024-S2029.

Donovan, D.C., Schingoethe, D.J., Baer, R.J., Ryali, J., Hippen, A.R.

and Franklin, S.T. (2000) Influence of dietary fish oil on conjugated linoleic acid and other fatty acids in milk fat from lactating dairy cows. *Journal of Dairy Science*, 83: 2620-2628.

Doreau, M., Chillard, Y., Rulquin, H. and Demeyer D.I. (1999) Manipulation of milk fat in dairy cows. in *Recent Advances in Animal Nutrition 1999*. P.C. Garnsworthy and J. Wiseman, eds. Nottingham University Press, Nottingham, UK.

Doreau, M. and Ferlay, A. (1994) Digestion and utilisation of fatty acids by ruminants. *Animal Feed Science and Technology*, 45: 379-396.

Drackley, J. K., Beaulieu, A.D. and Elliott, J.P. (2001) Responses of milk fat composition to dietary fat or nonstructural carbohydrates in Holstein and Jersey cows. *Journal of Dairy Science*, 84: 1231-1237.

Eastridge, M.L. and Firkins J.L. (2000) Feeding tallow triglycerides of different saturation and particle size to lactating dairy cows. *Animal Feed Science and Technology*, 83: 249-259.

Emery, R.S. (1978) Feeding for increased milk protein. *Journal of Dairy Science*, 61: 825-828.

Enjalbert, F., Nicot, M.C., Bayourthe, C., Vernay, M. and Moncoulon, R. (1997) Effect of dietary calcium salts of unsatuated fatty acids on digestion, milk composition and physical properties of butter. *Journal of Dairy Research*, 64: 181-195.

Erasmus, L.J., Hermansen, J.E. and Rulquin, E. (2001) Nutritional and management factors affecting milk protein content and composition. *International Dairy Federation Bulletin*, 366: 49-61.

Faverdin, P., Dulphy, J.P., Coulon, J.B., Vérité, R., Garel, J.P., Rouel, J. and Marquis B. (1991) Substitution of roughage by concentrates for dairy-cows. *Livestock Production Science*, 27: 137-156.

Ferlay, A., Martin, B., Pradel, P., Capitan, P., Coulon, J.B. and Chilliard, Y. (2002) Effect of the nature of forages on cow milk fatty acids having a positive role on human health. Pages 556-557 in *Multi-function grasslands: quality forages, animal products and landscapes*. Proceedings of the 19th General Meeting of the European Grassland Federation, 27-30 May 2002, La Rochelle, France.

Ferris, C.P., Gordon, F.J., Patterson, D.C., Kilpatrick, D.J., Mayne, C.S. and McCoy, M.A. (2001) The response of dairy cows of high genetic merit to increasing proportion of concentrate in the diet with a high and medium feed value silage. *Journal of Agricultural Science, Cambridge,* 136: 319-329.

Ferris, C.P., Gordon, F.J., Patterson, D.C., Mayne, C.S., and Kilpatrick, D.J. (1999) The influence of dairy cow genetic merit on the direct and residual response to level of concentrate supplementation. *Journal of Agricultural Science, Cambridge,* 132: 467-481.

Fitzgerald, J.J. and Murphy, J.J. (1999) A comparison of low starch maize silage and grass silage and the effect of concentrate supplementation of the forages or inclusion of maize grain with the maize silage on milk production by dairy cows. *Livestock Production Science*, **57**: 95-111.

Garnsworthy, P.C. (1996) The effects on milk yield and composition of incorporating lactose into the diet of dairy cows given protected fat. *Animal Science*, **62**: 1-3.

Garnsworthy, P.C. (1997) Fats in dairy cow diets. Pages 87-104 in *Recent Advances in Animal Nutrition 1997*. P. C. Garnsworthy and J. Wiseman, eds. Nottingham University Press, Nottingham, UK.

Garton, G.A. (1977) Fatty acid metabolism in ruminants. Pages 337-370 in *Biochemistry of Lipids II. Vol. 14*. T. W. Goodwin, ed. University Park Press, Baltimore.

Gasa, J., Holtenius, K., Sutton, J.D., Dhanoa, M.S. and Napper, D.J. (1991) Rumen fill and digesta kinetics in lactating dairy cows given two levels of concentrates with two types of grass silage ad lib. *British Journal of Nutrition*, **66**: 381-398.

Gerson, T., John, A., and King, A.S.D. (1985) The effect of dietary starch and fibre on the in vitro rates of lipolysis and hydrogenation by sheep rumen digesta. *Journal of Agricultural Science, Cambridge,* **105**: 27-30.

Gerson, T., John, A. and Sinclair, B.R. (1983) The effect of dietary N on in vitro lipolysis and fatty acid hydrogenation in rumen digesta from sheep fed diets high in starch. *Journal of Agricultural Science, Cambridge,* **101**: 97-101.

Givens, D.I. and Rulquin, H. (2002) Utilisation of protein from silage-based diets. Proceedings of the Eighth International Silage Conference, September 11-13th, Auchincriuve, Scotland, UK: 268-282.

Griinari, J.M. and Bauman D.E. (1999) Biosynthesis of conjugated linoleic acid and its incorporation into meat and milk in ruminants. Pages 180-200 in *Advances in conjugated linoleic acid research. Vol. 1*. M. P. Yurawecz, M.M. Mossoba, J.K.G., Kramer, M.W. Pariza, and G. Nelson, eds. AOCS Press.

Griinari, J.M., Bauman, D.E., and Jones, L.R. (1995) Low milk fat in New York Holstein herds. Pages 96-105 in Proceedings of the Cornell Nutrition Conference. Cornell University, Rochester, New York, USA.

Griinari, J.M., Corl, B.A., Lacy, S.H., Chouinard, P.Y., Nurmela, K.V.V. and Bauman, D.E. (2000) Conjugated linoleic acid is synthesized endogenously in lactating dairy cows by delta 9-Desaturase. *Journal of Nutrition*, **130**: 2285-2291.

Griinari, J.M., Dwyer, D.A., McGuire, M.A., Bauman, D.E., Palmquist, D.L. and Nurmela, K.V.V. (1998) *Trans*-octadecenoic acids and milk fat depression in lactating dairy cows. *Journal of Dairy Science*, **81**: 1251-1261.

Griinari, J.M., McGuire M.A., Dwyer D.A., Bauman D.E., Barbano

D.M., and House W.A. (1997) The role of insulin in the regulation of milk protein synthesis in dairy cows. *Journal of Dairy Science*, **80**: 2361-2371.

Griinari, M. and Shingfield, K.J. (2002) Effect of diet on trans fatty acids and conjugated dienes of linoleic acid in bovine milk fat. Proceedings of the 93rd Annual Meeting of the American Oil Chemists Society, Montreal, Canada, AOCS Press. S2.

Gordon, F.J. (1989) An evaluation through lactating cattle of a bacterial inoculant as an additive for grass silage. *Grass and Forage Science*, **44**: 169-179.

Grummer, R.R. (1991) Effect of feed on the composition of milk fat. *Journal of Dairy Science*, **74**: 3244-3257.

Gulati, S.K., May, C., Wynn, P.C. and Scott, T.W. (2002) Milk fat enriched in n-3 fatty acids. *Animal Feed Science and Technology*, **98**: 143-152.

Gunstone, F.D., Harwood, J.L. and Padley, F.B. (1994) Occurrence and characteristics of oils and fats. Pages 47-224 in *The Lipid Handbook*. Second ed. F.D. Padley, F.D. Gunstone, and J.L. Harwood, eds. Chapman and Hall, London, UK.

Gurr, M.I. (1999) Lipids in Nutrition and Health: A Reappraisal. No. 11. The Oily Press.

Ha, Y.L., Grimm, N.K. and Pariza, M.W. (1987) Anticarcinogens from ground beef: heat altered derivatives of linoleic acid. *Carcinogenesis*, **8**: 1881-1887.

Hanigan, M. D., B. J. Bequette, L. A. Crompton, and J. France. (2001) Modelling mammary amino acid metabolism. *Livestock Production Science*, **70**: 63-78.

Hanigan, M.D., Calvert, C.C., DePeters, E.J., Reis, B.L. and Baldwin, R.L. (1992) Kinetics of amino acid extraction by lactating mammary glands in control and sometribove-treated Holstein cows. *Journal of Dairy Science*, **75**: 161-173.

Hanigan, M. D., Cant, J.P., Weakly, D.C. and Beckett, J.L. (1998) An evaluation of postabsorptive protein and amino acid metabolism in the lactating dairy cow. *Journal of Dairy Science*, **81**: 3385-3401.

Harfoot, C. G. (1981) Lipid metabolism in the rumen. Pages 21-55 in *Lipid metabolism in ruminant animals*. W.W. Christie, ed. Pergamon Press Ltd., Oxford, UK.

Harfoot, C.G. and Hazlewood, G.P. (1997) Lipid metabolism in the rumen. Pages 382-426 in *The Rumen Microbial Ecosystem* (Second Edition). P.N. Hobson and D.S. Stewart, eds. Chapman and Hall, London, UK.

Harfoot, C.G., Noble, R.C. and Moore J.H. (1973) Food particles as a site for biohydrogenation of unsaturated fatty acids in the rumen. *Biochemical Journal*, **132**: 829-832.

Hawke, T.W. and Taylor J.C. (1995) Influence of nutritional factors on the yield, composition and physical properties of milk fat. Pages

37-88 in *Advanced Dairy Chemistry Volume 2: Lipids*. P. F. Fox, ed. Chapman and Hall, London, UK.

Hebeisen D.F., Hoeflin, F., Reusch, H.P., Junker, E. and Lauterburg, B.H. (1993) Increased concentrations of omega-3 fatty acids in milk and platelet rich plasma of grass-fed cows. International *Journal of Vitaminology and Nutrition Research*, **63**: 229-233.

Hegsted, D.M., McGandy, R.B. and Myers, M.L. (1965) Quantitative effects of dietary fat on serum cholesterol in man. *American Journal of Clinical Nutrition*, **17**: 281-295.

Henning, P.H., Steyen, D.G. and Meissner, H.H. (1993) Effect of synchronization of energy and nitrogen supply on ruminal characteristics and microbial growth. *Journal of Agricultural Science, Cambridge,* **73**: 142-148.

Hermansen, J.E. (1995) Prediction of milk fatty acid profile in dairy cows fed dietary fat differing in fatty acid composition. *Journal of Dairy Science*, **78**: 872-879.

Houssin, B., Foret, A. and Chenais, F. (2002) Effect of the winter diet (corn vs. grass silage) of dairy cows on the organoleptic quality of butter and camembert cheese. Pages 572-573 in *Multi-function grasslands: quality forages, animal products and landscapes*. Proceedings of the 19th General Meeting of the European Grassland Federation, 27-30 May 2002, La Rochelle, France.

Huhtanen, P. (1987) The effect of dietary inclusion of barley, unmolassed sugar- beet pulp and molasses on milk-production, digestibility and digesta passage in dairy-cows given silage based diet. *Journal of Agricultural Science, in Finland*, **59**: 101-120.

Huhtanen, P. (1988) The effects of barley, unmolassed sugar-beet pulp and molasses supplements on organic-matter, nitrogen and fiber digestion in the rumen of cattle given a silage diet. *Animal Feed Science and Technology*, **20**: 259-278.

Huhtanen, P. (1994) Forage influences on milk composition. Proceedings of Nova Scotia Forage Conference; Forage:Seeding to Feeding, The Nova Scotia Forage Council, Darthmouth, Nova Scotia, Canada (ed. A.F. Fredeen). 144-162.

Huhtanen, P. (1998) Supply of nutrients and productive responses in dairy cows given diets based on restrictively fermented silage. *Agricultural and Food Science in Finland*, **7**: 219-250.

Huhtanen, P., Jaakkola, S. and Saarisalo, E. (1995) The effects of concentrate energy-source on the milk-production of dairy-cows given a grass silage-based diet. *Animal Science*, **60**: 31-40.

Huhtanen, P., Miettinen, H. and Ylinen, M. (1993) Effect of increasing ruminal butyrate on milk yield and blood constituents in dairy cows fed a grass silage-based diet. *Journal of Dairy Science*, **76**: 1114-1124.

Huhtanen, P., Vanhatalo, A. and Varvikko, T. (2002) Effects of abomasal infusions of histidine, glucose, and leucine on milk production and plasma metabolites of dairy cows fed grass silage diets. *Journal of Dairy Science*, 85: 204-216.

Huhtanen, P.J., Blauwiekel, R. and Saastamoinen, I. (1998) Effects of intraruminal infusions of propionate and butyrate with two different protein supplements on milk production and blood metabolites in dairy cows receiving grass silage-based diet. *Journal of the Science of Food and Agriculture*, 77: 213-222.

Huntington, G.B. (1990) Energy metabolism in the digestive tract and liver of cattle: influence of physiological state and nutrition. *Reproduction, Nutrition Dévelopment*, 30: 35-47.

Huntington, G.B. (1997) Starch utilization by ruminants. From basics to the bunk. *Journal of Animal Science*, 75: 852-867.

Hurtaud, C., Delaby, L. and Peyraud, J. L. (2002a) Evolution of milk composition and butter properties during the transition between winter-feeding and pasture. Pages 574-575 in *Multi-function grasslands: quality forages, animal products and landscapes*. Proceedings of the 19th General Meeting of the European Grassland Federation, 27-30 May 2002, La Rochelle, France.

Hurtaud, C., Delaby, L. and Peyraud, J. L. (2002b) The nature of conserved forage affects milk composition and butter properties. Pages 576-577 in *Multi-function grasslands: quality forages, animal products and landscapes*. Proceedings of the 19th General Meeting of the European Grassland Federation, 27-30 May 2002, La Rochelle, France.

Hurtaud, C., Rulquin, H. and Verite, R. (1993) Effect of infused volatile fatty-acids and caseinate on milk- composition and coagulation in dairy-cows. *Journal of Dairy Science*, 76: 3011-3020.

Jaakkola, S. and Huhtanen P. (1993) The effects of forage preservation method and proportion of concentrate on nitrogen digestion and rumen fermentation in cattle. *Grass and Forage Science*, 48: 146-154.

Jacobs, J.L. and McAllan, A.B. (1992) Protein supplementation of formic acid and enzyme-treated silages. 2. Nitrogen and amino acid digestion. *Grass and Forage Science*, 47: 114-120.

Jenkins, T.C. (1993) Lipid metabolism in the rumen. *Journal of Dairy Science*, 76: 3851-3863.

Jenkins, T.C. (1998) Fatty acid composition of milk from Holstein cows fed oleamide or canola oil. *Journal of Dairy Science*, 81: 794-800.

Jenkins, T.C., Bateman, H.G. and Block, S.M. (1996) Butylsoyamide increases unsaturation of fatty acids in plasma and milk of lactating dairy cows. *Journal of Dairy Science* 79: 585-590.

Jensen, R.G. (2002) The composition of bovine milk lipids: January 1995 to December 2000. *Journal of Dairy Science*, 85: 295-350.

Jiang, J., Bjoerck, L., Fonden, R. and Emanuelson, M. (1996) Occurrence of conjugated *cis*-9, *trans*-11-octadecadienoic acid in bovine milk: Effects of feed and dietary regimen. *Journal of*

Dairy Science, **79**: 438-445.
Kalscheur, K.F., Teter, B.B., Piperova, L.S. and Erdman, R.A. (1997) Effect of fat source on duodenal flow of *trans*-$C_{18:1}$ fatty acids and milk fat production in dairy cows. *Journal of Dairy Science*, **80**: 2115-2126.
Karatzas, C.N. and Turner, J.D. (1997) Toward altering milk composition by genetic manipulation: Current status and challenges. *Journal of Dairy Science*, **80**: 2225-2232.
Keady, T.W.J. and Mayne C.S. (2001) The effects of concentrate energy source on feed intake and rumen fermentation parameters of dairy cows offered a range of grass silages. *Animal Feed Science and Technology*, **90**: 117-129.
Keady, T.W.J., Mayne, C.S., Fitzpatrick, D.A. and Marsden, M. (1999) The effects of energy source and level of digestible undegradable protein in concentrates on silage intake and performance of lactating dairy cows offered a range of grass silages. *Animal Science*, **68**: 763-777.
Keady, T.W.J., Mayne, C.S. and Marsden, M. (1998) The effects of concentrate energy source on silage intake and animal performance with lactating dairy cows offered a range of grass silages. *Animal Science*. **66**: 21-33.
Keady, T.W.J., Mayne, C.S. and Fitzpatrick, D.A. (2000) Effects of supplementation of dairy cattle with fish oil on silage intake, milk yield and milk composition. *Journal of Dairy Research*, **67**: 137-153.
Keady, T.W.J. and Murphy, J.J. (1996) Effects of inoculant treatment on ryegrass silage fermentation, digestibility, rumen fermentation, intake and performance of lactating dairy cattle. *Grass and Forage Science*, **51**: 232-241.
Keeney, M. (1970) Lipid metabolism in the rumen. Pages 489-503 in *Physiology of digestion and metabolism in the ruminant.* A. T. Phillipson, ed. Oriel Press, Newcastle-Upon-Tyne, UK.
Kelly, M.L., Kolver, E.S., Bauman, D.E., VanAmburgh, M.E. and Muller, L.D. (1998) Effect of intake of pasture on concentrations of conjugated linoleic acid in milk of lactating cows. *Journal of Dairy Science*, **81**: 1630-1636.
Kemp, P. and Dawson, R.M.C. (1968) Isomerization of linolenic acid by rumen micro-organisms. *Biochemial Journal*, **109**: 477-478.
Kemp, P. and Lander, D.J. (1984) Hydrogenation in vitro of alpha-linolenic acid to stearic acid by mixed cultures of pure strains of rumen bacteria. *Journal of General Microbiolgy*, **130**: 527-533.
Kennedy, J., Dillon P., Faverdin, P., Delaby, L., Buckley, F. and Rath, M. (2002) The influence of cow genetic merit for milk production on response to level of concentrate supplementation in a grass- based system. *Animal Science*, **75**: 433-445.
Kennelly, J.J. (1996) Producing milk with 2.5% fat-the biology and health implications for dairy cows. *Animal Feed Science and Technology*,

60: 161-180.

Kepler, C.R., Hirons, K.P., McNeill, J.J. and Tove, S.B. (1966) Intermediates and products of the biohydrogenation of linoleic acid by Butyrivibrio fibrisolvens. *Journal of Biological Chemistry*, 241: 1350-1354.

Keys, A.J.T., Anderson, F. and Grande, F. (1965) Serum cholesterol response to changes in the diet IV. Particularly saturated fatty acids in the diet. *Metabolism*, 14: 776-787.

Keys, A., Menotti, A., Karvonen, M.J., Aravanis, C., Blackburn, H., Buzina, R., Djordjevic, B.S., Dontas, A.S., Fidanza, F., and Keys, M.H. (1986) The diet and the 15-year death rate in the seven countries study. *American Journal of Clinical Epidemiology*, 124: 903-915.

Khalili, H. and Huhtanen, P. (1991) Sucrose supplements in cattle given grass silage based diet. 2. Digestion of cell wall carbohydrates. *Animal Feed Science and Technology*, 33: 262-273.

Kim, C. H., Choung, J.J. and Chamberlain, D.G. (1999) Determination of the first-limiting amino acid for milk production in dairy cows consuming a diet of grass silage and cereal-based supplement containing feather meal. *Journal of Science Food and Agriculture*, 79: 1703-1708.

Kim, C.H., Choung, J.J. and Chamberlain, D.G. (2000) The effects of intravenous administration of amino acids and glucose on the milk production of dairy cows consuming diets based on grass silage. *Grass and Forage Science*, 55: 173-180.

Kim, C.H., Kim, T.G., Choung, J.J. and Chamberlain, D.G. (2001) Effects of intravenous infusion of amino acids and glucose on the yield and concentration of milk protein in dairy cows. *Journal of Dairy Research*, 68: 27-34.

Kim, Y.J., Liu, R.H., Rychlik, J.L. and Russell, J.B. (2002) The enrichment of a ruminal bacterium (megasphaera elsdenii YJ-4) that produces the *trans*-10, *cis*-12 isomer of conjugated linoleic acid. *Journal of Applied Microbiology*, 92: 976-982.

Kinsella, J.E. (1972) Stearyl CoA as a precursor of oleic acid and glycerolipids in mammary microsomes from lactating bovine: possible regulatory step in milk triglyceride synthesis. *Lipids*, 7: 349-355.

Knekt, P., Jarvinen, R., Seppanen, R., Pukkala, E. and Aromaa, A. (1996) Intake of dairy products and the risk of breast cancer. *British Journal of Cancer*, 73: 687-691.

Knowlton, K.F., Dawson, T.E., Glenn, B.P., Huntington, G.B. and Erdman, R.A. (1998) Glucose metabolism and milk yield of cows infused abomasally or ruminally with starch. *Journal of Dairy Science*, 81: 3248-3258.

Korhonen, M., Ahvenjärvi, S., Vanhatalo, A. and Huhtanen, P. (2002) Supplementing barley or rapeseed meal to dairy cows fed grass-red clover silage: Amino acid profile of microbial fractions. *Journal* of *Animal Science*, **80**: 2188-2196.

Korhonen, M., Vanhatalo, A., Huhtanen, P. and Varvikko, T. (2000) Responses to graded postruminal doses of histidine in dairy cows fed grass silage diets. *Journal of Dairy Science*, **83**: 1-13.

Kowalski, Z.M., Pisulewski, P.M. and Spanghero, M. (1999) Effects of calcium soaps of rapeseed fatty acids and protected methionine on milk yield and composition in dairy cows. *Journal of Dairy Research*, **66**: 475-487.

Kritchevsky, D. (2000) Antimutagenic and some other effects of conjugated linoleic acid. *British Journal of Nutrition*, **83**: 459-465.

Lacasse, P., Kennelly, J.K., Delbecchi, L. and Ahnadi, C.E. (2002) Addition of protected and unprotected fish oil to diets for dairy cows. 1. Effects on the yield, composition and taste of milk. *Journal of Dairy Research*, **69**: 511-520.

Latham, M.J., Storry, J.E. and Sharpe, M.E. (1972) Effect of low-roughage diets on the microflora and lipid metabolism in the rumen. *Applied Microbiology*, **24**: 871-877.

Leaver, J.D. and Hill, J. (1995) The performance of dairy-cows offered ensiled whole-crop wheat, urea-treated whole-crop wheat or sodium hydroxide-treated wheat-grain and wheat-straw in a mixture with grass-silage. *Animal Science*, **61**: 481-489.

Lock, A.L. and Garnsworthy, P.C. (2002) Independent effects of dietary linoleic and linolenic fatty acids on the conjugated linoleic acid content of cows' milk. *Animal Science*, 74: 163-176.

Lock, A.L. and Garnsworthy P.C. (2003) Seasonal variation in milk conjugated linoleic acid and Delta(9)-desaturase activity in dairy cows. *Livestock Production Science* 79: 47-59.

Loor, J., Ferlay, A., Doreau, M. and Chilliard, Y. (2002a) Intestinal supply of *trans*-10, *cis*-12 conjugated linoleic acid lowers milk fat output in holstein cows fed a high- or low- fiber diet with two levels of linseed oil. *Journal of Dairy Science*, **85 (Suppl. 1)**: 297.

Loor, J.J. and Herbein, J.H. (1998) Exogenous conjugated linoleic acid isomers reduce bovine milk fat concentration and yield by inhibiting de novo fatty acid synthesis. *Journal of Nutrition*, **128**: 2411-2419.

Loor, J.J., Herbein, J.H. and Jenkins, T.C. (2002b) Nutrient digestion, biohydrogenation, and fatty acid profiles in blood plasma and milk fat from lactating Holstein cows fed canola oil or canolamide. *Animal Feed Science and Technology*, **97**: 65-82.

Mackle, T. R. and Bauman D.E. (1998) Recent developments in the regulation of milk protein production. Proceedings of the 1998 Cornell Nutrition Conference, Rochester, New York:104-112.

Mackle, T.R., Dwyer, D.A., Ingvartsen, K.L., Chouinard, P.Y., Lynch, J.M., Barbano, D.M. and Bauman, D.E. (1999) Effects of insulin and amino acids on milk protein concentration and yield from

dairy cows. *Journal of Dairy Science*, **82**: 1512-1524.
Mackle, T.R., Dwyer, D.A., Ingvartsen, K.L., Chouinard, P.Y., Ross, D.A. and Bauman, D.E. (2000) Effects of insulin and postruminal supply of protein on use of amino acids by the mammary gland for milk protein synthesis. *Journal of Dairy Science*, **83**: 93-105.
Maijala, K. (2000) Cow milk and human development and well-being. *Livestock Production Science*, **65**: 1-18.
Maniapane, E.H. and Salter, A.M. (1999) *Diet, lipoproteins and coronary heart disease: a biochemical perspective*. Nottingham University Press, Nottingham, UK.
Mansbridge, R.J. and Blake, J.S. (1997) Nutritional factors affecting the fatty acid composition of bovine milk. *British Journal of Nutrition*, **78**: S37-S47.
Martin, C., Bernard, L. and Michalet-Doreau, B. (1996) Influence of sampling time and diet on amino acid composition of protozoal and bacterial fractions from bovine ruminal contents. *Journal of Animal Science*, **74**: 1157-1163.
Martin, P.A., Chamberlain, D.G., Robertson, S. and Hirst, D. (1994) Rumen fermentation patterns in sheep receiving silages of different chemical-composition supplemented with concentrates rich in starch or in digestible fiber. *Journal of Agricultural Science, Cambridge,* **122**: 145-150.
Matitashvili, E., Baumgard, L.H. and Bauman, D.E. (2001) The effect of *trans*-10, *cis*-12 conjugated linoleic acid (CLA) infusion on milk fat synthesis and expression of lipogenic enzymes in the mammary gland of cows. *Journal of Dairy Science*, **84 (Suppl. 1)**: 310.
Mayne, C.S. (1990) An evaluation of an inoculant of Lactobacillus plantarum as an additive for grass silage for dairy cattle. *Animal Production*, **51**: 1-13.
Mayne, C.S. and Gordon, F.J. (1984) The effect of type of concentrate and level of concentrate feeding on milk-production. *Animal Production*, **39**: 65-76.
Mensink, R.P. and Katan, M.B. (1990) Effect of dietary trans fatty acids on high-density and low-density lipoprotein cholesterol levels in healthy subjects. *New England Journal of Medicine*, **323**: 439-445.
Mcguire, M.A., Griinari, J.M., Dwyer, D.A. and Bauman, D.E. (1995) Role of insulin in the regulation of mammary synthesis of fat and protein. *Journal of Dairy Science*, **78**: 816-824.
Mepham, T.B. (1976) The secretion of milk. *The Institute of Biology's Studies in Biology* (No. 60). The Camelot Press, Southampton, UK.
Mepham, T.B. (1982) Amino acid utilisation by the lactating mammary gland. *Journal of Dairy Science*, **65**: 287-298.
Mepham, T.B. (1987) Physiology of Lactation. Open University Press, Milton Keynes, UK.

Metcalf, J.A., Beever, D.E., Sutton, J.D., Wray-Cohen, D., Evans, R.T., Humphries, D.J., Blackwell, F.R.C, Bequette, B.J. and MacRae, J.C. (1994) The effect of supplementary protein on in vivo metabolism of the mammary gland in lactating dairy cows. *Journal of Dairy Science*, 77: 1816-1827.

Metcalf, J.A., Sutton, J.D., Cockburn, J.E., Napper, D.J., and Beever, D.E. (1991) The influence of insulin and amino-acid supply on amino-acid-uptake by the lactating bovine mammary-gland. *Journal of Dairy Science*, 74: 3412-3420.

Mettlin, C. and Graham S. (1979) Dietary risk factors in human bladder cancer. *American Journal of Epidemiology*, 110: 255-263.

Miettinen, H. and Huhtanen P. (1996) Effects of the ratio of ruminal propionate to butyrate on milk yield and blood metabolites in dairy cows. *Journal of Dairy Science*, 79: 851-861.

Miettinen, H. and Huhtanen P. (1997) Effects of silage fermentation and postruminal casein supplementation in lactating dairy cows. 2. Blood metabolites and amino acids. *Journal of the Science of Food and Agriculture*, 74: 459-468.

Molkentin, J. and Precht, D. (1995) Optimized analysis of *trans*-octadecenoic acids in edible fats. *Chromatographia*, 41: 267-272.

Moore, J.H. and Christie W.W. (1981) Lipid metabolism in the mammary gland of ruminant animals. Pages 227-277 in *Lipid metabolism in ruminant animals*. W. W. Christie, ed. Pergamon Press Ltd., Oxford, UK.

Mosley, E., Powell, G.L., Riley, M.B. and Jenkins, T.C. (2002) Microbial biohydrogenation of oleic acid to trans isomers in vitro. *Journal of Lipid Research*, 43: 290-296.

Murphy, J.J. (1986) A note on the use of pressed sugar-beet pulp in the diet of lactating dairy-cows. *Animal Production*, 43: 561-564.

Murphy, J.J. (2000) Synthesis of milk fat and opportunities for nutritional manipulation. British Society of Animal Science Occasional Publication Number, 25: 201-222.

Murphy, J.J. and O'Mara, F. (1993) Nutritional manipulation of milk protein concentration and its impact on the dairy industry. *Livestock Production Science*, 35: 117-134.

Ness, A.R., Smith, G.D. and Hart, C. (2001) Milk, coronary heart disease and mortality. *Journal of Epidemiology and Community Health*, 55: 379-382.

Newbold, J.R., Robertshaw, K.L. and Morris, H.W. (1998) Associations between concentrations of fat and intermediates of ruminal biohydrogenation in milk of dairy cows. *Proceedings of the British Society of Animal Science*, 224.

Noakes, M., Nestel, P.J. and Clifton, P.M. (1996) Modifying the fatty acid profile of dairy products through feedlot technology lowers plasma cholesterol of humans consuming the products. *American Journal of Clinical Nutrition*, 63: 42-46.

Noble, R.C. (1981) Digestion, transport and absorption of lipids. Pages 57-93 in *Lipid metabolism in ruminant animals*. W. W. Christie, ed. Pergamon Press Ltd., Oxford, UK.

Nocek, J.E. and Tamminga, S. (1991) Site of digestion of starch in the gastrointestinal-tract of dairy-cows and its effect on milk-yield and composition. *Journal of Dairy Science*, **74**: 3598-3629.

O'Donnell, J.A. (1989) Milk fat technologies and markets: a summary of the Wisconsin Milk Marketing Board 1988 milk fat roundtable. *Journal of Dairy Science*, **72**: 3109.

Offer, N.W., Marsden, M., Dixon, J., Speake, B.K. and Thacker, F.E. (1999) Effect of dietary fat supplements on levels of n-3 polyunsaturated fatty acids, trans acids and conjugated linoleic acid in bovine milk. *Animal Science*, **69**: 613-625.

Offer, N.W., Marsden, M. and Phipps, R.H. (2001b) Effect of oil supplementation of a diet containing a high concentration of starch on levels of trans fatty acids and conjugated linoleic acids in bovine milk. *Animal Science*, **73**: 533-540.

Offer, N.W., Speake, B.K., Dixon, J. and Marsden, M. (2001a) Effect of fish-oil supplementation on levels of (n-3) poly-unsaturated fatty acids in the lipoprotein fractions of bovine plasma. *Animal Science* **73**: 523–531.

Oldham, J.D. (1984) Protein-energy interrelationships in dairy cows. *Journal of Dairy Science*, **67**: 1090-1114.

O'Mara, F.P., Murphy, J.J., and Rath, M. (1997) The effect of replacing dietary beet pulp with wheat treated with sodium hydroxide, ground wheat, or ground corn in lactating cows. *Journal of Dairy Science*, **80**: 530-540.

O'Mara, F.P., Murphy, J.J. and Rath, M. (1998) Effect of amount of dietary supplement and source of protein on milk production, ruminal fermentation, and nutrient flows in dairy cows. *Journal of Dairy Science*, **81**: 2430-2439.

Onetti, S.G., Shaver, R.D., McGuire, M.A. and Grummer, R.R. (2001) Effect of type and level of dietary fat on rumen fermentation and performance of dairy cows fed corn silage-based diets. *Journal of Dairy Science*, **84**: 2751-2759.

Ørskov, E.R. and Reid, G.W. (1985) Use of by-products and supplementary protein in dairy cow nutrition. *Veterinary Record*, **116**: 607-610.

Overton, T.R., Cameron, M.R., Elliott, J.P., Clark, J.H. and Nelson, D.R. (1995) Ruminal fermentation and passage of nutrients to the duodenum of lactating cows fed mixtures of corn and barley. *Journal of Dairy Science*, **78**: 1981-1998.

Palmquist, D.L., Beaulieu, A.D. and Barbano, D.M. (1993) Feed and animal factors influencing milk fat composition. *Journal of Dairy Science*, **76**: 1753-1771.

Palmquist, D.L. and Jenkins, T.C. (1980) Fat in lactation rations: review. *Journal of Dairy Science*, **63**: 1-14.

Pariza, M.W., Ashoor, S.H., Chu, F.S. and Lund, D.B. (1979) Effects of temperature and time on mutagen formation in pan-fried hamburger. *Cancer Letters* 7: 63-66.

Parodi, P. W. (1994) Conjugated linoleic acid - an anticarcinogenic fatty acid present in milk fat. *Australian Journal of Dairy Technology*, 49: 93-97.

Parodi, P.W. (1997) Cows' milk fat components as potential anticarcinogenic agents. *Journal of Nutrition*, 127: 1055-1060.

Parodi, P.W. (1999) Conjugated linoleic acid and other anticarcinogenic agents of bovine milk fat. *Journal of Dairy Science*, 82:1339-1349.

Patterson, D.C., Yan, T., Gordon, F.J. and Kilpatrick, D.J. (1998) Effects of bacterial inoculation of unwilted and wilted grass silages. 2. Intake, performance and eating behaviour by dairy cattle. An evaluation of an inoculant/enzyme preparation as an additive for grass silage for cattle. *Journal of Agricultural Science, Cambridge*, 131: 113-119.

Perfield, J.W., Sæbø, A and Bauman, D.E. (2003) Effects of *trans*-8, *cis*-10 CLA and *cis*-11, *trans*-13 CLA on milk fat synthesis. American Dairy Science Association Annual Meeting, Phoenix, 2003 (in press).

Peterson, D.G., Baumgard, L.H. and Bauman, D.E. (2002) Short communication: Milk fat response to low doses of *trans*-10, *cis*-12 conjugated linoleic acid (CLA). *Journal of Dairy Science*, 85: 1764-1766.

Phipps, R.H., Sutton, J.D., Beever, D.E. and Jones, A.K. (2000) The effect of crop maturity on the nutritional value of maize silage for lactating dairy cows 3. Food intake and milk production. *Animal Science*, 71: 401-409.

Phipps, R.H., Sutton, J.D., Weller, R.F. and Bines, J.A. (1987) The effect of concentrate composition and method of silage feeding on intake and performance of lactating dairy-cows. *Journal of Agricultural Science, Cambridge,* 109: 337-343.

Piperova L.S., Sampugna, L., Teter, B.B., Kalscheur, K.F., Yurawecz, M.P., Ku, Y., Morehouse, K.M. and Erdman, R.A. (2002) Duodenal and milk trans octadecanoic acid and conjugated linoleic acid (CLA) isomers indicate that postabsorptive synthesis is the predominant source of *cis*-9-containing CLA in lactating dairy cows. *Journal of Nutrition,* 132: 1235-1241.

Piperova, L. S., Teter, B.B., Bruckental, I., Sampugna, J., Mills, S.E., Yurawecz, M.P., Fritsche, J., Ku, K. and Erdman, R.A. (2000) Mammary lipogenic enzyme activity, trans fatty acids and conjugated linoleic acids are altered in lactating dairy cows fed a milk fat-depressing diet. *Journal of Nutrition*, 130: 2568-2574.

Polan, C. E., Cummins, K.A., Sniffen, C.J., Muscato, T.V., Viciani, J.L., Crooker, B.A., Clark, J.H., Johnson, D.G., Otterby, D.E., Guillaume, B., Miller, L.D., Varga, G.A., Murray, R.A. and Peirce-

Sandner, S.B. (1991) Responses of dairy cows to supplemental rumen protected forms of methionine and lysine. *Journal of Dairy Science*, 74: 2997-3013.

Polan, C.E., McNeill, J.J. and Tove, S.B. (1964) Biohydrogenation of unsaturated fatty acids by rumen bacteria. *Journal of Bacteriology* 88: 1056-1064.

Poppitt, S.D., Keogh, G.F., Mulvey, T.B., McArdle, B.H., MacGibbon, A.K.H. and Cooper, G.J.S. (2002) Lipid-lowering effects of a modified butter fat: a controlled intervention trial in healthy men. *European Journal of Clinical Nutrition*, 56: 64-71.

Proell, J.M., Mosley, E., Powell, G.L. and Jenkins, T.C. (2002) Isomerization of stable isotopically labeled elaidic acid to cis and trans monoenes by ruminal microbes. *Journal of Lipid Research*, 43: 2072-2076.

Reynolds, C.K., Cammell, S.B., Humphries, D.J., Beever, D.E., Sutton, J.D. and Newbold, J.R. (2001) Effects of postrumen starch infusion on milk production and energy metabolism in dairy cows. *Journal of Dairy Science* 84: 2250-2259.

Reynolds, C.K., Harmon, D.L., and Cecava M.J. (1994) Absorption and delivery of nutrients for milk protein-synthesis by portal-drained viscera. *Journal of Dairy Science*, 77: 2787-2808.

Reynolds, C.K., Sutton, J.D. and Beever, D.E. (1997) Effects of feeding starch to dairy cattle on nutrient availability and production. Pages 105-134 in *Recent Advances in Animal Nutrition 1997*. P. C. Garnsworthy and J. Wiseman, eds. Nottingham University Press, Nottingham, UK.

Ridsig, R.B. and Schultz L.H. (1974) Effects of abomasal infusions of safflower oil or eladic acid on blood lipids and milk fat in dairy cows. *Journal of Dairy Science*, 57: 1459-1466.

Rinne, M., Jaakkola, S., Varvikko, T. and Huhtanen, P. (1999a) Effects of type and amount of rapeseed feed on milk production. *Acta Agriculturae Scandinavica Section A-Animal Science*, 49: 137-148.

Rinne, M., Jaakkola, S., Kaustell, K., Heikkilä, T. and Huhtanen, P. (1999b) Silages harvested at different stages of growth v. concentrate foods as energy and protein sources in milk production. *Animal Science* 69: 251-263.

Robinson, P.H. (1996) Rumen protected amino acids for dairy cattle: what is the future? *Animal Feed Science and Technology*, 59: 81-86.

Romney, D.L., Blunn V., Sanderson, R., and Leaver, J.D. (2000) Feeding behaviour, food intake and milk production responses of lactating dairy cows to diets based on grass silage of high or low dry-matter content, supplemented with quickly and slowly fermentable energy sources. *Animal Science*, 71: 349-357.

Rook, J.A. and Balch, C.C. (1961) The effects of intraruminal infusions of acetic, propionic and butyric acids on the yield and composition of the milk of the cow. *British Journal of Nutrition*, 15: 361-369.

Rook, J.A., Balch, C.C. and Johnson, V.W. (1965) Further observations on the effects of intraruminal infusions of volatile fatty acids and lactic acid on the yield and composition of the milk of the cow. *British Journal of Nutrition*, **19**: 93-99.

Rooke, J.A., Lee, N.H. and Armstrong, D.G. (1987) The effects of intraruminal infusions of urea, casein, glucose syrup and a mixture of casein and glucose syrup on nitrogen digestion in the rumen of cattle receiving grass-silage diets. *British Journal of Nutrition*, **57**: 89-98.

Rulquin, H. (1982) Effects sur la digestion et le metabolisme des vaches laitieres d'infusions d'acides gras volatils dans le rumen et de caseinate dans le duodenum. 1. Production et digestion. *Reproduction, Nutrition, Dévelopment*, **22**: 905-921.

Rulquin, H., Pisulewski P. M., Vérité R., and Guinard J. (1993) Milk production and composition as a function of postruminal lysine and methionine supply: a nutrient-response approach. *Livestock Production Science*. **37**: 69-90.

Rulquin, H. and Vérité R. (1993) Amino acid requirements of dairy cows: productive effects and animal requirements. Page 55-65 in *Recent Advances in Animal Nutrition* 1993. P.C. Garnsworthy and D.J.A. Cole, eds. Nottingham University Press, Nottingham, UK.

Sanderson, P., Gill, J.M.R., Packard, C.J., Sanders, T.A.B., Vessby, B. and Williams, C.M. (2002) UK food standards agency *cis*-monounsaturated fatty acid workshop report. *British Journal of Nutrition*, **88**: 99-104.

Samuelson, G., Bratteby, L.E., Mohsen, R., and Vessby, B. (2001) Dietary fat intake in healthy adolescents: inverse relationships between the estimated intake of saturated fatty acids and serum cholesterol. *British Journal of Nutrition,* **85**: 333-341.

Satter, L.D. (1986) Protein supply from undegraded dietary protein. *Journal of Dairy Science*, **69**: 2734-2749.

Santos, F.A.P., Santos, J.E.P., Theurer, C.B. and Huber, J.T. (1998) Effects of rumen-undegradable protein on dairy cow performance: A 12-year literature review. *Journal of Dairy Science*, **81**: 3182-3213.

Schwab, C.G., Bozak, C.K., Whitehouse, N.L. and Mesbah, M.M.A. (1992) Amino acid limitation and flow to duodenum at four stages of lactation. 1. Sequence of lysine and methionine limitation. *Journal of Dairy Science*, **75**: 3486-3502.

Schwab, C.G., Satter, L.D. and Clay, A.B. (1976) Response of lactating dairy cows to abomasal infusion of amino acids. *Journal of Dairy Science*, **59**: 1254-1270.

Seal, C.J. and Reynolds, C.K. (1993) Nutritional implications of gastrointestinal and liver metabolism in ruminants. *Nutrition Research Reviews*, **6**: 185-208.

Shingfield, KJ. (2000) Estimation of microbial protein supply in ruminant animals based on renal and mammary purine metabolite excretion. A review. *Journal of Animal and Feed Sciences*, **9**: 169-212.

Shingfield, K.J., Ahvenjärvi, S., Toivonen, V., Ärölä, A., Nurmela, K. V. V., Huhtanen, P. and Griinari, J.M. 2003a. Effect of fish oil on biohydrogenation of fatty acids and milk fatty acid content. Animal Science *77*: 165-179.

Shingfield, K.J., Vanhatalo, A. and Huhtanen. P. 2003b. Comparison of heat-treated rapeseed expeller and solvent-extracted soyabean meal protein supplements on the performance of dairy cows fed grass silage-based diets. Animal Science *77*: 305-317.

Shingfield, K.J., Jaakkola, S. and Huhtanen, P. (2002a) Effect of forage conservation method, concentrate level and propylene glycol on diet digestibility, rumen fermentation, blood metabolite concentrations and nutrient utilisation of dairy cows. *Animal Feed Science and Technology*, **97**: 1-21.

Shingfield, K.J., Jaakkola S. and Huhtanen, P. (2002b) Effect of forage conservation method, concentrate level and propylene glycol on intake, feeding behaviour and milk production of dairy cows. *Animal Science*, **74**: 383-397.

Shingfield, K.J., Jaakkola S. and Huhtanen, P. (2001) Effects of level of nitrogen fertilizer application and various nitrogenous supplements on milk production and nitrogen utilization of dairy cows given grass silage-based diets. *Animal Science*, **73**: 541-554.

Siddons, R.C., Nolan, J.V., Beever, D.E. and Macrae, J.C. (1985) Nitrogen digestion and metabolism in sheep consuming diets containing contrasting forms and levels of N. *British Journal of Nutrition*, **54**: 175-187.

Sinclair, L.A., Garnsworthy, P.C., Newbold, J.R. and Buttery, PJ. (1993) Effect of synchronizing the rate of dietary energy and nitrogen release on rumen fermentation and microbial protein synthesis in sheep. *Journal of Agricultural Science, Cambridge,* **120**: 251-263.

Sloan, B.K. (1997) Developments in amino acid nutrition of dairy cows. Pages 167-198 in *Recent Advances in Animal Nutrition 1997*. P. C. Garnsworthy and J. Wiseman, eds. Nottingham University Press, Nottingham, UK.

Sloan, B.K., Rowlinson P., and Armstrong D.G.. (1988) Milk-production in early lactation dairy-cows given grass- silage ad-libitum - influence of concentrate energy-source, crude protein-content and level of concentrate allowance. *Animal Production*, **46**: 317-331.

Smedman, A., Gustafsson, I.B., Berglund, L. and Vessby, B. (1999) Pentadecanoic acid (C15:0) in serum as a marker for intake of milk fat. The relationships between the intake of milk fat and metabolic risk factors. *American Journal of Clinical Nutrition*, **69**: 22-29.

Spörndly, E. (1989) Effects of diet on milk composition and yield of dairy cows with special emphasis on milk protein content. Swedish

Journal of Agricultural Research, **19**: 99-106.
Storry, J.E. (1981) The effect of dietary fat on milk composition. Pages 3-34 in *Recent Advances in Animal Nutrition 1981*. W. Haresign, ed. Butterworths, London, UK.
St Pierre, N.R. (2001) Invited review: Integrating quantitative findings from multiple studies using mixed model methodology. *Journal of Dairy Science*, **84**: 741-755.
Steinmetz, K.A., Childs, M.T., Stimson, C., Kushi, L.H., McGovern, P.G., Potter, J.D., and Yamanaka ,W.K. (1994) Effect of consumption of whole milk and skim milk on blood lipid profiles in healthy men. *American Journal of Clinical Nutrition*, **59**:612-618.
Stern, M.D. (1986) Efficiency of microbial protein synthesis in the rumen. Pages 10-19 in Proceedings of the 1986 Cornell Nutrition Conference for Feed Manufacturers. Ithaca, NY, USA.
Sutton, J.D. (1989) Altering milk composition by feeding. *Journal of Dairy Science*, **72**: 2801-2814.
Sutton, J.D., Abdalla, A.L., Phipps, R.H., Cammell, S. B. and Humphries, D.J. (1997) The effect of the replacement of grass silage by increasing proportions of urea-treated whole-crop wheat on food intake and apparent digestibility and milk production by dairy cows. *Animal Science*, **65**: 343-351.
Sutton, J.D., Broster, W.H., Schuller, E., Napper, D.J., Broster, V.J. and Bines, J.A. (1988) Influence of plane of nutrition and diet composition on rumen fermentation and energy-utilization by dairy-cows. *Journal of Agricultural Science, Cambridge,* **110**: 261-270.
Sutton, J.D., Cammell, S.B., Beever, D.E., Humphries, D.J. and Phipps, R.H. (1998) Energy and nitrogen balance of lactating dairy cows given mixtures of urea-treated whole-crop wheat and grass silage. *Animal Science*, **67**: 203-212.
Sutton, J.D., Cammell, S.B., Phipps, R.H., Beever, D.E. and Humphries, D.J. (2000) The effect of crop maturity on the nutritional value of maize silage for lactating dairy cows 2. Ruminal and post-ruminal digestion. *Animal Science*, **71**: 391-400.
Sutton, J.D., Morant, S.V., Bines, J.A., Napper, D.J. and Givens, D.I. (1993) Effect of altering the starch - fiber ratio in the concentrates on hay intake and milk-production by friesian cows. *Journal of Agricultural Science, Cambridge,* **120**: 379-390.
Sutton, J.D., Phipps, R.H., Deaville, E.R., Jones, A.K. and Humphries, D.J. (2002) Whole-crop wheat for dairy cows: effects of crop maturity, a silage inoculant and an enzyme added before feeding on food intake and digestibility and milk production. *Animal Science*, **74**: 307-318.
Sutton, J. D., Storry J E., and Nicholson J. W. (1970) The digestion of fatty acids in the stomach and intestines of sheep given widely different rations. *Journal of Dairy Research*, **37**: 97-105.

Syrjälä, L. (1972) Effect of different sucrose, starch and cellulose supplements on the utilization of grass silages by ruminants. *Annales Agriculturae Fenniae* 11: 199-276.

Tamminga, S. (2001) Effects of feed, feed composition and feed strategy on fat content and fatty acid composition in milk. *International Dairy Federation Bulletin*, **366**: 15-27.

Tesseraud, S., Grizard, J., Makarski, B., Debras, E., Bayle, G. and Champredon, C. (1992) Effect of insulin in conjunction with glucose, amino-acids and potassium on net metabolism of glucose and amino-acids in the goat mammary-gland. *Journal of Dairy Research*, **59**: 135-149.

Theurer, C.B., Huber J.T., Delgado-Elorduy A. and Wanderley, R. (1999) Invited review: Summary of steam-flaking corn or sorghum grain for lactating dairy cows. *Journal of Dairy Science*, **82**: 1950-1959.

Tholstrup, T., Sandstrom, B., Hermansen, J.E. and Hølmer, G. (1998) Effect of modified dairy fat on postprandial and fasting plasma lipids and lipoproteins in healthy young men. *Lipids*, **33**: 11-21.

Thomas, C. (1987) Factors affecting substitution rates in dairy cows on silage based rations. Pages 205-218 in *Recent Advances in Animal Nutrition 1987*. W. Haresign and D.J.A. Cole, eds. Butterworths, London.

Thomas, C., Aston, K., Daley, S.R. and Bass, J. (1986) Milk-production from silage 4. The effect of the composition of the supplement. *Animal Production*. **42**: 315-325.

Thomas, C. and Rae R.C.. (1988) Concentrate supplementation of silage for dairy cows. Pages 327-354 in *Nutrition and Lactation in the Dairy Cow*. P. C. Garnsworthy, ed. Butterworth, London, UK.

Thomas, P.C. and Chamberlain, D.G. (1982) Silage as a foodstuff. Pages 63-101 in *Silage for Milk Production, Technical Bulletin 2*. J. A. Rook and P. C. Thomas, eds. NIRD-HRI.

Thomas, P.C. and Chamberlain, D.G. (1984) Manipulation of milk composition to meet market needs. Pages 219-243 in *Recent Advances in Animal Nutrition*. W. Haresign and D. J. A. Cole, eds. Butterworths, London, UK.

Thomas, P.C. and P.A. Martin. (1988) The influence of nutrient balance on milk yield and composition. Pages 97-118 in Nutrition and Lactation in *the Dairy Cow*. P. C. Garnsworthy, ed. Butterworths, London, UK.

Thomas, P.C. and S. Robertson. (1987) The effect of lipid and fibre source and content on silage intake, milk production and energy utilisation. Proceedings of the Eighth Silage Conference, Hurley: 173-174.

Tuori, M. (1992) Rapeseed meal as a supplementary protein for dairy-cows on grass silage-based diet, with the emphasis on the nordic aat- pbv feed protein evaluation system. *Agricultural Science in*

Finland, 1: 375-429.

Van Vuuren, A.M., Klop, A., Van der Koelen, C.J., and De Visser, H. (1999) Starch and stage of maturity of grass silage: Site of digestion and intestinal nutrient supply in dairy cows. *Journal of Dairy Science*, **82**: 143-152.

Vanhatalo, A., Huhtanen, P., Toivonen, V. and Varvikko, T. (1999) Response of dairy cows fed grass silage diets to abomasal infusions of histidine alone or in combinations with methionine and lysine. *Journal of Dairy Science*, **82**: 2674-2685.

Varvikko, T., Vanhatalo, A., Jalava, T. and Huhtanen, P. (1999) Lactation and metabolic responses to graded abomasal doses of methionine and lysine in cows fed grass silage diets. *Journal of Dairy Science*, **82**: 2659-2673.

Viswanadha, S., Hanson, T.W., Giesy, J.G. and McGuire, M.A. (2000) Response of milk fat to intravenous administration of the *trans*-10, *cis*-12 isomer of conjugated linoleic acid (CLA). *Journal of Dairy Science*, **83 (Suppl. 1)**: 163.

Volden, H. and Harstad, O.M. (1998) Amino acid composition of bacteria harvested from the rumen of dairy cows fed three diets differing in protein content and rumen protein degradability at two levels of intake. *Acta Agriculturae. Scandinavica, Section A, Animal Science*, **48**: 210-215.

Volden, H., Mydland, L.T. and Harstad, O.M. (1999) Chemical composition of protozoal and bacterial fractions isolated from ruminal content of dairy cows fed diets differing in nitrogen supplementation. *Acta Agriculturae. Scandinavica, Section A, Animal Science*, **49**: 235-244.

Wall, R.J., Kerr, D.E. and Bondioli, K.R. (1997) Transgenic dairy cattle: Genetic engineering on a large scale. *Journal of Dairy Science*, **80**: 2213-2224.

Wilde, P.F. and Dawson, R.M.C. (1966) The biohydrogenation of alpha-linolenic acid and oleic acid by rumen micro-organisms. *Biochemical Journal*, **98**: 469-475.

White, S.L., Bertrand, J.A., Wade, M.R., Washburn, S.P., Green, J.T. and Jenkins, T.C. (2001) Comparison of fatty acid content of milk from Jersey and Holstein cows consuming pasture or a total mixed ration. *Journal of Dairy Science*, **84**: 2295-2301.

Whitelaw, F.G., Milne, J.S., Ørskov, E.R. and Smith, J.S. (1986) The nitrogen and energy metabolism of lactating cows given abomasal infusion of casein. *British Journal of Nutrition*, **55**: 537-556.

Williams, C.M. (2000) Dietary fatty acids and human health. *Annales de Zootechnie*, **49**:165-180.

Willett, C.W., Stampfer, M.J., Manson, J.E., Colditz, G.A., Speizer, F.E., Rosner, B.A., Sampson, L.A. and Hennekens, C.H. (1993) Intake of trans fatty acids and risk of coronary heart disease among women. *Lancet*. **341**: 581-585.

Wiseman, M.J. (1997) Fat and fatty acids in relation to cardiovascular disease: an overview. *British Journal of Nutrition*, 78 (Suppl. 1): S3-S4.

Wolff, R.L. and Bayard, C.C. (1995) Improvement in the resolution of individual *trans*-18/1 isomers by capillary gas-liquid-chromatography - use of a 100-m CP-Sil-88 column. *Journal of the American Oil Chemists Society*, 72: 1197-1201.

Wu, Z. and Huber, J.T. (1994) Relationship between dietary-fat supplementation and milk protein-concentration in lactating cows - a review. *Livestock Production Science*, 39: 141-155.

Zerbini, E., Polan, C.E. and Herbein, J.H. (1988) Effect of dietary soybean meal and fish meal on protein digesta flow in Holstein cows during early and midlactation. *Journal of Dairy Science*, 71: 1248-1258.

Zock, P.L. and Katan, M.B. (1997) Trans fatty acids, lipoproteins and coronary risk. *Canadian Journal of Physiology and Pharmacology*, 75: 211-216.

6

USING BIOTECHNOLOGY FOR THE PRODUCTION AND ENHANCEMENT OF LIVESTOCK FEED

Gary F. Hartnell
Monsanto Company, 800 N Lindbergh Blvd, St. Louis, MO, 63167, U.S.A

Introduction

The human race has previously utilized biotechnology (defined as the use of microorganisms or biological substances to perform industrial purposes) for thousands of years to produce foods such as beer, wine, cheese and yogurt. In recent decades, biotechnology has been successfully employed to improve plant and animal products beneficial to livestock and humans while indirectly improving the environment through pesticide reduction. Since the late 1970's, biotechnology has incorporated the use of genetic engineering and recombinant DNA technology. Through the adoption of these new techniques, a purer source of insulin was produced in 1982 which is the main commercial source used today taking the place of animal-derived insulin. In 1983, the first genetically modified plant was produced followed in 1990 by transgenic production of enzymes used for cheese production. Today, biotechnology touches the food, feed, beverage and pharmaceutical industries as well as others. Genetically enhanced feed and food crops in U.S. include maize, canola, cotton, rice, tomatoes, potatoes, and soybeans. Peppers, sunflowers, and peanuts are in the pipeline for approval. Other genetically engineered feed and food crops such as sugar beets, wheat, squash, papayas, berries, bananas, and pineapples, have been developed in laboratories and will head for marketing within the next few years. Biotechnology keys will open doors to future processes and products benefiting the environment, animals and mankind in ways that are dreams today (Hartnell, 2001).

Currently, more than 50 million hectares are planted globally with biotech crops, primarily with agronomic qualities to improve yield through resistance to insect damage, tolerance to herbicides used to control weeds and protection from viruses (James, 2002). Crop producers experience direct benefits through increased yields and reduced production costs with these modified agricultural commodities. Whether for agricultural or other purposes, transgenic traits are currently being evaluated for their potential to: 1) protect plants against insect damage, fungal, viral, or bacterial diseases; 2) provide selective tolerance to herbicides used for weed control; 3) enhance crop yields; 4) increase nutritional quality and health benefits to animals and humans; 5) reduce naturally occurring toxicants or allergens; 6) modify the ripening process and provide superior flavor; 7) utilize plants as factories to make products such as biodegradable polymers or pharmaceutical products; 8) modify food composition for disease prevention. Advances in genetics and new technologies are producing feeds and foods with greater yields to meet the needs of a growing world population. Nonetheless, development and commercialization of biotechnology products are being debated.

Safety and risks

World Health Organization, Food and Drug Administration, and other government and international scientific organizations have considered the risks and have concluded that plant biotechnology does not pose any unique risk compared with other production methods (FAO/WHO, 1991). As with human food safety assessment, the safety assessment of a novel livestock feed looks at the compositional, toxicological, and nutritional characteristics of the biotech feed in comparison with its conventional counterpart. This assessment includes the source of the gene, molecular characterization of the gene; history and safe use of the expressed protein, protein function, concentration, toxicology and mode of action; crop agronomic characteristics; and composition. For example, insect-protected proteins isolated from *Bacillus thuringiensis* (Bt) have been registered for use as microbial insecticides since 1961. The microbial Bt formulations contain Cry insect proteins (Cry is an acronym for crystalline protein inclusions) that have an exemplary safety record following 40 years of use in agriculture (Betz, Hammond and Fuchs, 2000). Organic farmers in the U.S. have been and are using microbial Bt formulations for insect control. There are currently at least 180 registered microbial Bt products in the U.S. (EPA, 1998b). Following a single acute exposure, Cry proteins bind to specific receptors in the midgut cells of susceptible insects and form ion-selective channels in the cell membrane (English and Slatin, 1992). The cells swell due to an influx of water that leads to cell lysis, the insect stops eating and dies (Knowles and Ellar, 1987). If receptor binding does not occur, the Cry protein has no effect on that organism. Mammals do not have Cry protein specific bindings sites on intestinal epithelial cell membranes (Noteborn, Rienenmann-Ploum, van der Berg, Alink, Zolla and Kuiper, 1994; Hofmann, Luthy, Hutter and Pliska, 1988). This explains why the Cry insect control proteins are acutely toxic to target insects at mg/kg body weight doses, but are non-toxic to mammals dosed acutely with greater than 1×10^6 mg/kg Cry insect control proteins (EPA 1998a; McClintock, Schaffer and Sjoblad, 1995).

All commercially approved transgenic products containing insect protection or herbicide tolerance traits are substantially equivalent to their conventional counterparts. In addition, nutritional equivalence has been further demonstrated in numerous livestock feeding studies conducted globally with no unintended effects (Aumaitre, Aulrich, Chesson, Flachowsky and Piva, 2002; Clark and Ipharraguerre, 2001; Flachowsky and Aulrich, 2001, Hartnell, Stanisiewski and Glenn, 2002). There are over 100 references in the literature reporting results and/or reviewing studies covering the feeding of crops containing insect-protected and/or herbicide-tolerant traits to animals (poultry, swine, beef cattle, dairy cattle, sheep, water buffalo, fish, and rabbits) all concluding nutritional equivalence (see http://www.animalbiotechnology.org).

Consumer groups have asked whether direct human consumption of the DNA or protein in plant biotech products impacts human health and whether human consumption of animal products (e.g. meat, milk or eggs) from farm animals fed the biotech crops are safe. The United Nations FAO and WHO (1991), the U.S. FDA (1992) and the U.S. EPA (2000) have each stated very clearly that the consumption of DNA from all sources – including plants improved through biotechnology– is safe, given the long history of safe consumption of DNA. Beever and Kemp (2000) and Beever and Phipps (2001) have discussed the *in vivo* fate of DNA and concluded that there is a growing body of scientifically valid information available indicating no significant risk associated with the consumption of DNA or resulting proteins from GM crops. Even though DNA (plant, animal, microbial, etc.) has been consumed from the beginning of mankind and deemed safe, studies were conducted in attempt to detect the transgenic DNA in milk, meat and eggs. Also, measurement of transgenic protein was attempted in these same tissues in spite of their rapid digestion in the gut and proven safety. All studies confirmed that transgenic proteins and DNA could not be detected in meat, milk or eggs (Hartnell *et al.*, 2002). Over six years of feeding transgenic crops to livestock in the US has further confirmed the safety of these products with no unintended effects.

Risks of releasing GM crops into the environment are outside the scope of this paper. However, some recent reviews have been written that cover the issues in detail (CAST, 1999; Conner, Glare and Nap, 2003; Nap, Metz, Esclaer and Conner, 2003; NAS, 2002).

Nutritional benefits for livestock

Through biotechnology, the livestock industry will have the opportunity to select crops as feed ingredients that optimize performance and profits for their specific enterprise. Precision gene insertion through recombinant technology now enables one to up-regulate or down-regulate specific metabolic pathways or insert new pathways in plants resulting in enhanced protein quality and/or quantity, modified amino acid levels (i.e., high lysine maize), modified carbohydrate composition and content (i.e., starch, oil, cellulose, hemicellulose, pectin), reduced lignin, reduced indigestible oligosaccharide content, increased levels of oligofructans, enhanced vitamin content, and incorporation of natural compounds for improved feed efficiency and growth performance (Araba, 1997; Bajjalieh, 1996, Owens and Sonderlund, 2000; Parsons, Zhang and Araba, 2000; Sauber, 2000). High oleic acid soybean will provide high energy concentrations. Grains with oligofructans may reduce the need for antibiotics. The transformation of active components found in botanicals into crops may offer a future substitute for antimicrobials.

Halpin, Foxon and Fentem (1995) reviewed transgenic approaches for manipulating the starch biosynthesis, sucrose accumulation, fructan biosynthesis and seed oil content in crops. The amount and type of starch is very important for driving rumen fermentation in ruminants and meeting energy needs of monogastrics. Increasing the proportion of oil in corn grain is important in increasing the energy density of the grain. These non-structural carbohydrate components are all important for enhancing value to the livestock.

Producers may have the ability to select specific grains or protein sources that were designed for optimizing performance and profitability of their particular livestock enterprise. White and Higgins (2000) reported an eight percent increase in wool growth and seven percent increase in live weight gain in sheep fed modified lupin. Lupin was genetically modified to contain a sunflower gene that produces a protein that is both rich in sulfur amino acids and stable in the sheep's rumen.

Stock (1999) reviewed the effects of nutritional changes in cereal grains from genetic modification in beef feedlot diets. One of the earliest examples of genetic manipulation was the introduction of tannins into grain sorghum hybrids to decrease losses from birds and preharvest mold. The beneficial change also resulted in decreased digestibility of the grain. Efforts continue to improve digestibility without sacrificing grain yield, drought or heat tolerance. Data on the evaluation of waxy corn, high lysine corn, high oil corn and other grains in beef feedlot diets is limited. Results to date are variable.

Stilborn (1999) recently examined the future of designer grains for nonruminants. Benefits from feeding high oil corn (HOC) to broilers may include a reduction in abdominal fat and increased breast meat yield when diets contain similar nutrient to energy ratios as the yellow corn control diets. HOC may be used to increase the energy intake of the laying hen during peak production. In swine diets, HOC can be used to either increase dietary energy density or replace yellow dent corn and supplemental fat. Nutritional inputs to consider include high lysine and/or high methionine high oil corn, high lysine, methionine or protein in corn and soybean meal with high lysine or methionine concentrations. High oleic acid, high oil corn will offer livestock producers the ability to modify the fatty acid profile of lipid deposited in the carcass resulting in improved processing, storage and consumer preference properties.

Nutritional value of genetically improved high lysine, high oil corn was evaluated in young pigs (O'Quinn, Nelssen, Goodband, Knabe, Woodworth, Tokach and Lohrmann, 2000). Researchers reported the lysine in the high lysine, high corn was as available as that in the high oil corn based on results of a pig digestibility and a performance trial. High lysine, high oil corn offers the potential to reduce the amount of supplemental protein and/or lysine and energy needed in swine diets.

Future opportunities associated with biotechnology could lead to transfer of traits to meat, milk and or eggs which produce products such as anti-cancer agents, anti-oxidants, anti-aging agents, health enhancing agents, natural meat tenderizers, modified fatty acid products, and disease preventive agents.

Safer and quality-enhanced feed

Insect-protected plants that have been commercialized are genetically enhanced to produce *in planta* insect control proteins similar to those produced by the soil bacterium *Bacillus thuringiensis* (*Bt*). Research has consistently demonstrated significant reductions in total fumonisin (B1, B2 and B3) concentrations in maize kernels containing the Cry1Ab protein when the hybrids were infested with European Corn Borer (Dowd, 2000; Munkvold, Hellmich and Rice, 1999). A safer maize supply will result in reduced incidence of mycotoxicosis (fumonisin) in livestock.

Genetically modifying crops to contain mannanoligosaccharide or enhancing yeasts to produce more mannanoligosaccharides for feeding may benefit animal health and performance. Recent research has shown the supplementation of the diet with modified mannanoligosaccharide to be beneficial in counteracting the adverse effects of dietary mycotoxins on the immunological status of broiler breeder hens (Afzali and Devegowda, 1999) and significantly improving body weight, feed consumption and antibody titers in broilers (Raju and Devegowda, 1999).

Development of crops having low or no anti-nutritional factors will benefit animals and producers through improved digestibility and nutrient utilization. Biotechnology is the best tool currently available to plant scientists to reduce or eliminate undesirable components of feed ingredients such as erucic acid and glucosinolates in rapeseeds; trypsin inhibitor, lectin, raffinose and stachyose in soybean; tannin in sorghum; glucosinolates in cotton; and protease inhibitors, phytohemagglutinins, and cyanogens and bloat compounds in legumes in a timely fashion.

Animal health

Plants have considerable potential for production of biopharmaceutical proteins and peptides including edible vaccines that can be stored and distributed as seeds, tubers, or fruits (Giddings, Allison, Brooks and Carter, 2000). In particular, the chicken interferon gene is being incorporated into corn so a particular protein can be produced in the seed as a vaccine to help combat avian influenza and help keep chickens healthy. The market (estimated $1.7 billion USD market for chicken vaccines) is high because farmers who raise the world's 18 billion chickens live in fear of the outbreak of virulent avian influenza strains. ProdiGene (College Station, Texas) received a patent covering viral disease vaccines produced in genetically enhanced plants (Feedstuffs, Vol. 71, 1999). The vaccines produced via this technology can be marketed either in edible form, made from parts of the fruit, vegetable or grain plant or in injectable form. Hepatitis B in humans and transmissible gastroenteritis virus (TGV) in swine are two diseases being targeted. Clinical trials for the TGV vaccines are underway. Other oral vaccines under development for swine include vaccines against porcine reproductive and respiratory syndrome (PRRS) and diseases like parvovirus (http://agbio.cabweb.org/news/research.htm).

Environmental benefits

Livestock producers will continue to face issues regarding livestock waste management including waste disposal, excessive phosphorus and nitrogen excretion, methane production and odor. Increasing digestibility of nutrients in animal feeds will be a major factor in reducing livestock waste problems. In the future, forages will be bioengineered to contain more digestible fiber components and/or fiber digestive enzymes. The plant may contain lignin, cellulose and hemicellulose that are more easily degraded or cellulase, hemicellulase and lignase enzymes may be bioengineered into plants or rumen microbes that enhance the utilization of these energy sources. Low lignin corn is already here via plant breeding. The brown mid rib mutant gene was identified and bred into certain lines of corn. This product contains about 40% less lignin than its parental variety. Enzymes could be genetically engineered to convert roughages to substrates now utilizable by monogastrics.

Microbes (silage microbial innoculants) could be genetically modified to enhance the fermentation process of forages in silos. Feedstuffs will have more balanced amino acid patterns, more digestible carbohydrate components and optimum fatty acid profiles.

Mineral bioavailability will be improved to make more efficient use of the minerals in plants and reduce the contribution to the environment where leaching can occur in streams and lakes. Phosphorus is the main mineral of concern at this time. Phosphorus is locked up in the plant as phytate phosphorus. Monogastric animals do not have the necessary enzyme machinery to access the phosphorus so it ends up in animal waste. The waste is applied to the fields where leaching and run-off can occur. To prevent this problem phytase enzyme is added to poultry and swine feed to unlock this valuable mineral (Stilborn, 1999). Through biotechnology, plants will contain low phytate (high available phosphorus) or phytase activity thus allowing for more efficient use of phosphorus with reduced supplementation of inorganic sources and (Stilborn, 1999).

Bioengineered crops may be developed resulting in reduced animal wastes, greenhouse gases and less offensive manure odors.

Conclusion

Recombinant DNA technology is producing revolutionary changes in agriculture. With the adoption of biotechnology, food and feeds will be more abundant, more nutritious, more stable in storage, safer, and healthier than current foodstuffs. The fruits of agricultural biotechnology will also include an improved environment for humans and livestock producers as foods are produced using less pesticides and herbicides. Improved animal efficiency and feed digestibility will result in less animal wastes. Biotechnology must be considered as an important tool for sustaining agriculture to meet the demands of the world's rapidly increasing population for now and the future.

References

Afzali, N. and Devegowda, G. (1999) Ability of modified mannanoligosaccharide to counteract aflatoxicosis in broiler breeder hens. *Poultry Science,* 78 (Suppl. 1), 52.

Araba, M. (1997) Impact of new grain varieties on feed manufacturing. *Feed Management*, 48 (1), 11.

Aumaitre, A., Aulrich, K., Chesson, A., Flachowsky, G. and Piva, G. (2002) New feeds from genetically modified plants: substantial equivalence, nutritional equivalence, digestibility, and safety for animals and the food chain. *Livestock Production Science*, 74, 223-238.

Bajjalieh, N.L. (1996) Added-value grains to have expanded value in feed. *Feedstuffs*, 68, 23.

Betz, F.S., Hammond, B.G. and Fuchs, R.L. (2000) Safety and advantages of *bacillus thuringiensis*-protected plants to control insect pests. *Regulatory Toxicology and Pharmacology*, 32, 156-173.

Beever, D.E. and Kemp, C.F. (2000) Safety issues associated with the DNA in animal feed derived from genetically modified crops. A review of scientific and regulatory procedures. *Nutrition Abstracts and Reviews, Series B, Livestock Feeds and Feeding*, 70 (3), 175-182.

Beever, D.E. and Phipps, R.H. (2001) The fate of plant DNA and novel proteins in feeds for farm livestock: A United Kingdom perspective. *Journal of Animal Science*, 79, E290-E295.

CAST (Council for Agriculture Science and Technology). (1999) *Applications of Biotechnology to Crops: Benefits and Risks*. Issue Paper 12, Ames, Iowa, USA: CAST(http://www.cast-science.orgpdfbiotc_ip.pdf).

Clark, J.H. and Ipharraguerre, I.R. (2001) Livestock performance: Feeding Biotech crops. *Journal of Dairy Science*, 84 (E. Suppl.), E9-E18.

Conner, A.J., Glare, T.R. and Nap, J. (2003) The release of genetically modified crops into the environment. Part II. Overview of ecological risk assessment. *The Plant Journal*, 33, 19-46.

Dowd, P. (2000) Indirect reduction of era molds and associated mycotoxins in *Bacillus thuringiensis* corn under controlled and open field conditions: utility and limitations. *Journal of Economic Entomology*, 93, 1669-1679.

English, L. and Slatin, S.L. (1992) Mode of action of delta-endotoxin from *Bacillus thuringiensis*: a comparison with other bacterial toxins. *Insect Biochemistry and Molecular Biology*, 22, 1-7.

EPA. (1998a). EPA Registration Eligibility Decision (RED) *Bacillus thuringiensis*. EPA 738-R-98-004, March 1998.

EPA. (1998b). (RED Facts) *Bacillus thuringiensis*. EPA-738-F-98-001.

FAO/WHO. (1991) Strategies for assessing the safety of foods produced by biotechnology. Report of a Joint FAO/WHO Consulation. Food and Agriculture Org/World Health Org. World health Org., Geneva.

Flachowsky, G. and Aulrich, K. (2001) Nutritional assessment of feeds from genetically modified organism. *Journal of Animal and Feed Science*, 10 (Suppl. 1), 181-194.

Giddings, G., Allison G., Brooks D. and Carter, A. (2000) Transgenic plants as factories for biopharmaceuticals. *Nature Biotechnology*, 18, 1151-1155.

Halpin, C., Foxon, G.A. and Fentem, P.A. (1995) Transgenic plants with improved energy characteristics. *In Biotechnology in Animal Feeds and Animal Feeding,* pp. 279-293. Edited by R.J. Wallace and A. Chesson. VCH Publishers, New York, USA.

Hartnell, G.F. (2001) Futuristic aspects of biotech food for livestock and humans. *In Midwest Swine Nutrition Conference Proceedings, Indianapolis, Indiana, September 5, 2001*, pp 47-57.

Hartnell, G.F., Stanisiewski, E.P. and Glenn, K.C. (2002) Feed safety and performance of livestock fed biotech enhanced crops. *Proceedings of California Animal Nutrition Conference, Fresno, USA, May 8 and 9, 2002*, pp 9-28.

Hofmann, C., Luthy, P., Hutter, R. and Pliska, V. (1988) Binding of the delta endotoxin from *Bacillus thuringiensis* to brush-border membrane vesicles of the cabbage butterfly (*Pieris brassicae*). *European Journal of Biochemistry*, **173**, 85-91.

James, C., (2002) Global review of commercialized transgenic crops: 2001. ISAAA Briefs No. 24: Preview.

Knowles, B.H. and Ellar, D.J. (1987) Colloid-osmotic lysis is a general feature of the mechanisms of action of *Bacillus thuringiensis* (delta)-endotoxins with different insect specificity. *Biochemical and Biophysical Acta,* **924**, 509-518.

McClintock, J.T., Schaffer, C.R. and Sjoblad, R.D. (1995) A comparative review of the mammalian toxicity of *Bacillus thuringiensis*-based pesticides. *Pesticide Science*, **45**, 95-105.

Munkvold, G.P., Hellmich, R.L. and Rice, L.G. (1999) Comparison of fumonisin concentrations in kernels of transgenic Bt maize hybrids and nontransgenic hybrids. *Plant Dispersal,* **83**, 130-138.

Nap, J., Metz, P.L.J., Escaler, M. and Conner, A.J. (2003) The release of genetically modified crops into the environment. Part I. Overview of current status and regulations. *The Plant Journal*, **33**, 1-18.

NAS (National Academy of Aciences). (2002) *Environmental Effects of Transgenic Plants: the Scope and Adequacy of Regulation.* Washington D.C.: National Academy Press (http://books.nap.edu/books/0309082633/html/index.html).

Noteborn, H.P.J.M., Rienenmann-Ploum, M.E., van den Berg, J.H.J., Alink, G.M., Zolla, L. and Kuiper, H.A. 1994. Consuming transgenic food crops: the toxicological and safety aspects of tomato expressing Cry1Ab and NPTII. ECB6: *Proceeding of the 6th European Congress on biotechnology*, Elsevier Science.

O'Quinn, P.R., Nelssen, J.L., Goodband, R.D., Knabe, D.A., Woodworth, J.C., Tokach, M.D. and Lohrmann, T.T. (2000) Nutritional value of a genetically improved high-lysine, high-oil corn for young pigs. *Journal of Animal Science,* **78**, 2144

Owens, F. and Soderlund, S. (2000) Specialty Grains for Ruminants. 61th Minnesota Nutrition Conference & Minnesota Soybean Research and Promotion Council Technical Symposium, September

19-20, 2000, Bloomington, MN. Conference Proceedings p 98-113.2149.

Parsons, C.M., Zhang Y. and Araba, M. (2000) Nutritional evaluation of soybean meals varying in oligosaccharide content. *Poultry Science,* 79, 1127-1131.

Raju, M.V.L.N. and Devegowda, G. (1999) Influence of modified mannanoligosaccharide on broilers exposed to individual and combined mycotoxicoses of aflatoxin, ochratoxin and T-2 toxin. *Poultry Science,* 78 (Suppl. 1), 52.

Sauber, T. (2000) Performance of Soybean Meals Produced From Genetically Enhanced Soybeans. *61st Minnesota Nutrition Conference & Minnesota Soybean Research and Promotion Council Technical Symposium, September 19-20, 2000, Bloomington, USA, Conference Proceedings* pp 44-51.

Stilborn, H.L. (1999) The future of designer grains for non-ruminants. *60th Minnesota Nutrition Conference & ZinPro Technical Symposium, September 20-22, 1999 Bloomington, USA, Conference Proceedings,* p 144.

Stock, R.A. (1999) Nutritional benefits of specialty grain hybrids in beef feedlot diets. *Journal of Dairy Science* 82(Suppl 2), 208 or *Journal of Animal Science* 77(Suppl 2), 208.

U.S. EPA. (2000) Biopesticides Registration Action Document: Bt Plant-Pestdicides, October 18-20.

U.S. Food and Drug Administration. (1992) Statement of Policy: Foods Derived from New Plant Varieties, *Notice, Federal Register,* 57, 104. 22984-23005.

7

MILK, BLOOD LIPIDS AND CORONARY HEART DISEASE (CHD) - 'THE MYTH AND THE EVIDENCE'

Anne M. Minihane
Hugh Sinclair Unit of Human Nutrition, School of Food Biosciences, University of Reading, Reading RG6 6AP, UK

Introduction

Chronic diet related diseases such as cardiovascular disease (CVD) and cancers account for the vast majority (~ 65%) of total mortality in the UK (Figure 1). In westernised countries average life expectancy is rapidly increasing with the ratio of people of working age to people over 65 estimated to fall from about to 4:1 to 2.5:1 by the year 2040. These ageing population demographics have placed an almost unbearable strain on the health care systems of these countries. As a result there has been increased focus on the use of diet as a modifiable means of preventing or delaying the onset of disease. This approach in addition to being cost effective would ensure that for the individual who is living longer that they also remain healthier for longer, developing chronic life threatening diseases at an older age.

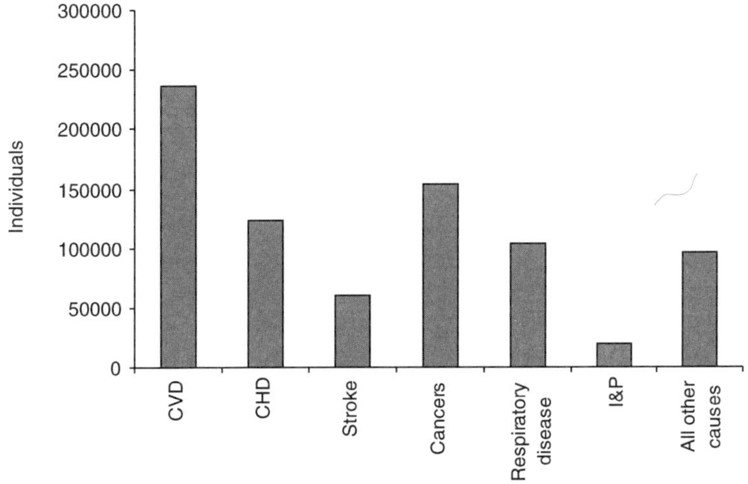

Figure 1. Causes of death in the UK (2000) (Adapted from Office for National Statistics, 2001). Keys to abbreviations are: CVD- Cardiovascular disease, CHD- Coronary Heart Disease and I&P- Injuries and Poisoning.

With respect to CVD the dietary focus has been on the fat content of the diet, with a reduction in total and saturated fat recommended to lower disease incidence. As dairy products contribute up to 20% and 40% of total fat and saturated fat respectively in the UK diet, much recent attention has focussed on the association between the consumption of dairy products in particular milk products and the risk of disease. The public perception of dairy products and the evidence linking this source of fat to the occurrence of CVD will be considered.

Fat profile of bovine milk

The fat composition of bovine milk is variable, with season, and the diet and breed of the animal impacting on the fatty acid profile. The typical composition of whole and reduced fat milk and yoghurt is given in Table 1 and Figure 2. Approximately 60% of bovine milk fat is saturated (SFA) in nature with 25% existing as monounsaturated fatty acids (MUFA). Over 65% of the total SFA content is present as lauric acid (C12:0), myristic acid (C14:0), or palmitic acid (C16:0) which are the important fatty acids with respect to blood cholesterol levels (see later).

Table 1. Typical fatty acid profile of a selection of milk products. (Adapted from McCance and Widdowson, 1998)

Fatty acid g/100g food	*Whole milk*	*Semi-skimmed milk*	*Yogurt (whole milk)*	*Yogurt (low fat)*
Total Fat	4.0	1.7	3.0	1.0
Total SFA	2.48	1.07	1.91	0.66
Total MUFA (*cis*)	0.93	0.39	0.71	0.23
Total PUFA (*cis*)	0.10	0.04	0.07	0.03
Total *trans*	0.14	0.07	0.05	0.01
C4:0	0.14	0.06	0.11	0.04
C6:0	0.09	0.04	0.07	0.02
C8:0	0.05	0.02	0.04	0.01
C10:0	0.11	0.05	0.08	0.02
C12:0	0.15	0.07	0.12	0.03
C14:0	0.41	0.18	0.32	0.10
C16:0	1.06	0.46	0.82	0.30
C18:0	0.41	0.18	0.31	0.11
C18:1-*cis*	0.79	0.34	0.61	0.19
Trans MUFA	0.01	tr	0.08	0.02
C18:2-*cis* (n-6)	0.07	0.01	0.05	0.03
C18:3-*cis* (n-6)	0	0	0	0
C20:4-*cis* (n-6)	0	0	0	0
C18:3-*cis* (n-3)	0.02	0.01	0.02	tr
C20:5-*cis* (n-3)	0	0	0	0
C22:5-*cis* (n-3)	tr	tr	0	0
C22:6-*cis* (n-3)	0	0	0	0
Total *trans* PUFA	0.03	0.02	0.03	Tr

SFA- saturated fatty acids, MUFA- monounsaturated fatty acids, PUFA- polyunsaturated fatty acids

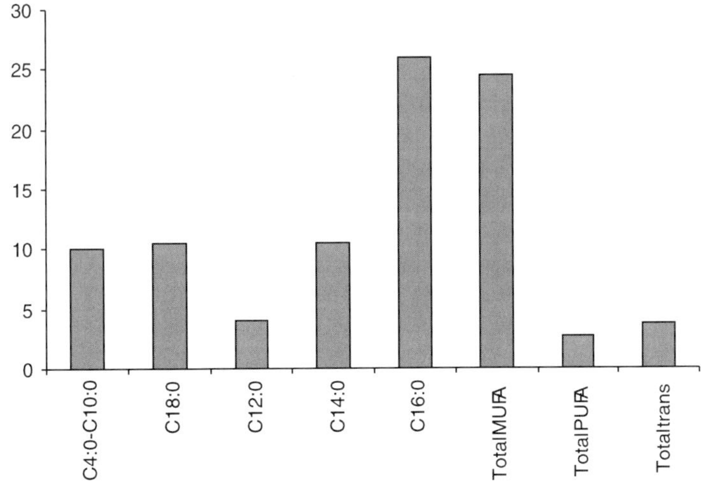

Figure 2. The fatty acid composition of bovine milk fat. Keys to abbreviations are: MUFA- monounsaturated fatty acids, PUFA- polyunsaturated fatty acids, and trans- trans fatty acids

A popular misconception which exits is that all saturated fats in the diet come from animal products such as milk and that all vegetable oils contain only MUFA and polyunsaturated fatty acids (PUFA). Although many vegetable oils such as corn oil, sunflower oil and olive oil are rich sources of these fatty acids, oils such as coconut oil and palm oil, which are commonly added to processed foods contain 80-90% SFA.

The trans fatty acid (TFA) content of bovine fat lies somewhere between 2-5% of total fat, with vaccenic acid being the primary trans fatty acid present (Figure 3). The other major dietary source of TFA are those formed during the hydrogenation of vegetable oils in order to provide a more solid fat source. Between 5-25% of the total fat of hydrogenated vegetable oils are in the TFA form, although recent focus on the negative impact of TFA on CVD risk has resulted in significant decreases in the TFA content of processed foods. The association between TFA from different sources and CVD incidence will be given later.

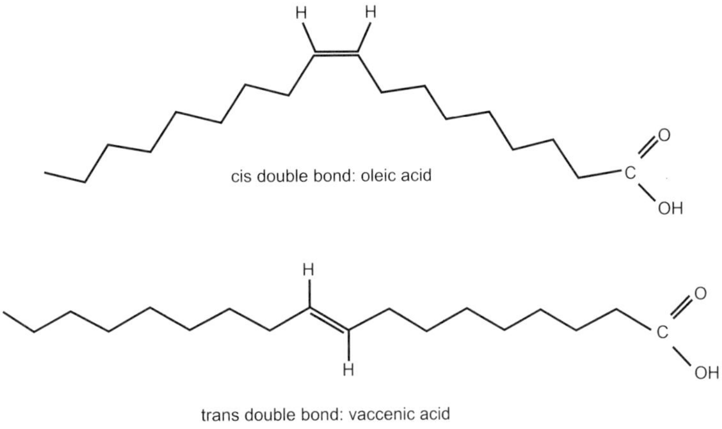

Figure 3. Structure of *trans* fatty acids

Cardiovascular disease

Cardiovascular disease (CVD) refers to diseases of the heart and circulatory system and includes both coronary heart disease (CHD) and stroke. In the UK, CVD is the main cause of death, accounting for over 235,000 deaths in 2000 (Figure 1), with over one in three people (39%) dying from the condition. The risk of developing CVD is determined by a number of non-modifiable and modifiable risk factors with diet and in particular dietary fat arguably the most important modifiable environmental risk factor.

The primary pathological features underlying CVD are atherosclerosis and thrombosis. Atherosclerosis is a thickening and narrowing of the arteries ('furring'), caused by a build up of plaque in the inner artery wall (intima), which usually occurs in large and medium-sized arteries. This plaque is made up of cholesterol, muscle cells, fibrous tissue, calcium and clumps of platelets. Plaques may grow large enough to significantly reduce the blood flow through a particular vessel. In addition the plaque may rupture which may stimulate the blood to clot (thrombosis). The combination of narrowing of the artery and a blood clot in an artery supplying the heart muscle (coronary artery) can cause oxygen deprivation and a build up of waste in the heart tissue supplied by that particular vessel, which can result in a heart attack. If a blood vessel supplying the brain is blocked, it can cause a stroke

Lipid hypothesis and cardiovascular disease

Atherosclerosis is a complex chronic condition, which begins in childhood. The lipid hypothesis exemplifies the role of raised levels of blood lipids in the development of atherosclerosis and CHD. Whilst historically blood cholesterol was considered to be the only important blood lipid (cholesterol hypothesis) with high circulating levels associated with increased disease risk, recent evidence suggests that the circulating levels of triglycerides (TG) are also an important determinant of disease risk.

Lipid transport

Cholesterol and triglycerides cannot dissolve in the blood and have to be transported in special particles called lipoproteins. Lipoproteins are protein (apolipoprotein), lipid (cholesterol, triglyceride, phospholipids) complexes which may be broadly divided into four main categories. Chylomicrons and very low density lipoproteins (VLDL) transport fat from the small intestine (dietary fat) or fat formed in the liver, to the target cells where it can be used immediately as a source of fuel or as a building block for a range of important cell compounds. Excess fat is stored as a reserve in the adipose tissue. Low-density lipoproteins (LDL) represent the main form of cholesterol in the circulation, with on average 70% of total cholesterol being present as LDL. LDL is formed from the degradation of VLDL. The majority of cholesterol deposited in the artery wall during the progression of atherosclerosis is derived from LDL and it is therefore commonly referred to as 'bad cholesterol'. In contrast high-density lipoproteins (HDL)- cholesterol is referred to as 'good cholesterol'. HDL is the particle responsible for the transport of excess cholesterol, from the body tissues, including the artery walls, back to the liver. High levels of HDL are therefore cardioprotective.

Cholesterol hypothesis

Evidence for the involvement of cholesterol in the development of CHD began with the recognition of waxy deposits in the arteries of cholesterol-fed rabbits at the turn of the last century (Anitshkow, 1913), and culminated in a recent series of randomly controlled clinical intervention trials which demonstrated that cholesterol-lowering drugs can reduce the risk of death from CHD (Scandinavian Simvastatin Survival Study Group, 1994; Shepherd, Cobbe, Ford, Isles, Lorimer, MacFarlane and Packard, 1995). Levels of cholesterol in the blood, specifically LDL-cholesterol are now arguably recognised as the most important physiological determinant of CHD risk with a reduction of 1% associated with a 2% reduction in risk. It has been estimated that 40-50% of deaths from coronary heart disease (CHD) in the UK are due to a raised cholesterol level (above 5.2mmol/l).

As a result a vast array of pharmacological and dietary intervention designed to delay atherogenesis focus on normalising cholesterol levels in the blood.

Triglycerides and CHD

However not all people who suffer a heart attack have elevated cholesterol levels. It is vital to remember that the aetiology of CHD is multifactorial and other risk factors are also important in disease progression. Circulating levels of trigylcerides are now recognised as a significant independent risk marker for CHD (Hokanson and Austin, 1996). Triglycerides containing particles, in particular chylomicron and VLDL remnants can infiltrate and transport fat into the artery wall. Furthermore high levels of TG are associated with a lowering in HDL-cholesterol and an increase in the proportion of LDL as LDL-3, which is the form of LDL which most rapidly accumulates in the artery wall.

Dietary fats and blood lipids

It has been almost 40 years since Keys, Anderson and Grande (1965) published their initial findings from the *'Seven Countries Cohort Study'*. This landmark study marked the beginning of our understanding of the association between dietary fat and blood lipid levels with the total fat, saturated fat and polyunsaturated fats recognised as important determinants of circulating cholesterol levels. Since then numerous epidemiological and intervention studies have contributed to our knowledge and although the findings are not always consistent the main conclusions are as follows (Mensink and Katan, 1992; Hegsted, Ausman, Johnson and Dallal, 1993).

- Increased total dietary fat increases LDL-cholesterol and TG levels.
- Saturated fatty acids are a primary determinant of LDL-C. However not all SFA behave the same. The shorter chain SFA (less than 12 carbon atoms) and stearic acid (C18:0) are thought to be relatively neutral. It is mainly lauric acid (C12:0), myristic acid (C14:0) and palmitic acid (C16:0) which are the hypercholesterolaemic SFA.
- Replacement of dietary SFA with n-6 PUFA and MUFA results in a reduction in LDL-C.
- All fatty acids increases HDL-C levels when they replace carbohydrate in the diet with SFA being the most effective.
- Since the early 1990's much media attention has focussed on the deleterious impact of *trans* fatty acids (TFA). Vaccenic acid from ruminal products (i.e. milk and meat), and a range of TFA formed during industrial hydrogenation, in particular, elaidic acid are the primary TFA's in the diet (Figure 3). Early studies suggested that this group of fatty acids had a potent negative effect on blood lipids, resulting in a significant increase in total- and LDL-cholesterol and a decrease in HDL-cholesterol. However in these earlier intervention trials, intakes of TFA of between 10-20% of dietary energy were assessed, levels of intake far in excess of habitual intakes in the UK (<2% dietary energy). More recent studies, suggest a less dramatic effect on lipoprotein metabolism, with Mensink and Zock (1998) concluding in a recent meta-analysis that each 1% increase in dietary energy from TFA results in an 0.028mmol/l (< 1%) increase in LDL-C. Furthermore it appears that not all TFA behave the same. In the Nurses Health Study, a large prospective study involving 85,000 women, an increased risk of CHD was observed at the highest intake of TFA (Willett, Stampfer, Manson, Colditz, Speizer, Rosner, Sampson and Hennekens, 1993)(Table 2). A subsequent subgroup analysis demonstrated that the increased CHD risk was only associated with *trans* isomers from hydrogenated vegetable fats as found in spreads, cakes and biscuits, whereas no association was found with the TFA in dairy products. Although the issue remains contentious, it is likely that the current intakes of TFA from milk and dairy products and

meat in the UK has a minimal impact on blood lipid levels and CHD risk.

Table 2. Relative risk of coronary heart disease in relation to *trans* fatty acid intake in women.

	RR in quintiles					
	1	*2*	*3*	*4*	*5*	*P*
Total *trans* isomers	1.0	1.23	1.11	1.36	1.67	0.002
Isomers from vegetable sources	1.0	1.43	1.11	1.39	1.78	0.009
Isomers from animal sources	1.0	0.76	0.69	0.55	0.59	0.230

365 cases of CHD with participants divided into quintiles on the basis of *trans* fatty acid intake. The data is adjusted for energy intake, dietary lipids, smoking, body mass index, hypertension, alcohol intake, menopausal status, postmenopausal oestrogen use, family history of myocardial infarctions before the age of 60, and multivitamin use. Adapted from Willett *et al.* (1993).

- The cardioprotective benefits of the long chain n-3 PUFA fish oil fatty acids, eicosapentaenoic acid (EPA) and docosahexaenoic acid (DHA) are well documented. In addition to a range of other benefits a intake of 2-4g per day have been shown to reduce TG levels by up to 35% with an associated increase in HDL-cholesterol (Minihane, Khan, Leigh-Firbank, Talmud, Wright, Murphy, Griffin and Williams, 2000).
- Much recent attention has focussed on the benefits of conjugated linoleic acid (CLA). Milk and dairy products are the almost exclusive dietary source of these group of 18-carbon unsaturated fatty acid derivatives, with intakes in the UK estimated to be 0.1-0.2g/day. However, data on CLA is limited, with high dietary intakes been shown to delay the progression of atherosclerosis in animal models (Kritchevsky, Tepper, Wright, Tso and Czarnecki, 2000). Data on the impact of CLA on blood lipids and the progression of atherosclerosis in humans is distinctly lacking. Extrapolation from animal studies suggest that intakes > 100-fold higher than the current intakes may be necessary to bring about any benefit with respect to CHD incidence in humans (Williams, 2000). The data is most promising with respect to its anti-carcinogenic action, with the c9, t-11 CLA isomer shown to protect against the development of chemically induced cancers in experimental animals (Ha, Storkson and Pariza, 1990). Although data is limited a small number of epidemiological studies also suggest that CLA may offer some protection against breast cancer development in humans (Knekt, Jarvinen, Seppanen, Pukkala and Aromaa, 1996).

Milk fat and CHD-the 'myths'

The myth that modest intakes of milk are associated with increased CHD incidence and mortality are based around two misconceptions. Firstly that milk is a high fat product. In a survey conducted by the National Dairy Council UK in 1997 (Figure 4), 1000 members of the public were questioned on the total fat content of milk products. On average individuals considered whole milk, semi-skimmed and skimmed milk to contain 32%, 15% and 8% fat respectively which is far removed from the true values of less than 4%, 2% and 0.2% respectively. Although dairy products contribute up to 20% of total fat intake in the UK (16g fat), only a small fraction of this is consumed as milk. An intake of 0.5 litre of milk per day, would only increase total fat intake by 2g, which would represent < 3g of total dietary fat. The second misconception is that milk, by virtue of its fatty acid composition, with about 60% of the total fat present as saturated fat, is often viewed as having the potential to elevate blood cholesterol levels and therefore exert an adverse effect of cardiovascular health. However evidence to substantiate such a suggestion is distinctly lacking as will be discussed

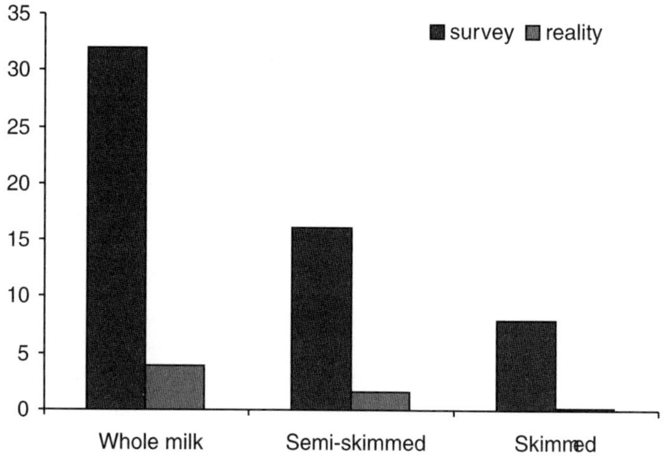

Figure 4. Public perception of fat in milk.

Milk fat and CHD-the 'evidence'

Epidemiological data and findings from dietary intervention studies examining the contribution of milk consumption to blood cholesterol and CHD incidence is limited and conflicting.

Epidemiological evidence

The epidemiological findings linking milk consumption and CHD can be unrealiable, due to the inaccuracies of dietary assessment techniques, and the contribution of confounding factors to the outcomes. In the Seven Coutries Study associations between 18 different food groups and 25-year mortality from CHD was investigated in 16 cohorts spanning 7 countries (Menotti Kromhout, Blackburn, Fidanza, Buzina and Nissinen, 1999). A positive univariate between total animal fat and milk intake and CHD death was observed. A study by Hu, Rimm, Stampfer, Ascheiro, Spiegelman and Willett (2000) notes a strong positive association between a "Western Pattern" diet which included red meat, processed meat, sweets and desserts, french fries and dairy products was evident. However the individual effect of milk was not evaluated. In contrast to the findings of the Seven Countries Cohort Study, the West of Scotland Prospective Study observed no relationship between the consumption of whole milk and cardiovascular death. (Ness, Smith and Hart, 2001). Information on the amount of milk consumed was obtained from a single question issued to 5,765 men between 1970 and 1973. Over the next 25 years the study recorded 1,212 deaths from cardiovascular disease, but could find no relationship with milk consumption. On the contrary, moderate milk consumption (190-750ml/day) was actually found to be associated with a reduced risk (-8%) of CHD death. The investigators acknowledge the fact that milk drinkers had healthier lifestyles and a more favourable socio-economic status than the non-milk drinkers, the latter of which were likely to be shorter, older, heavier consumers of alcohol and smokers. Nevertheless, the association with reduced CHD risk was still maintained even after adjustment for these factors with an adjusted relative risk (RR) of 0.93 (95% CI 0.83-1.04) in moderate consumers, rising to 0.64 (95% CI 0.4-1.0) in men with higher intakes (>750ml/day). Even if this potentially beneficial effect was ignored, the authors claim that it is highly unlikely that the study would have failed to detect a positive relationship between milk consumption and CHD, if it existed in this high-risk population.

Randomly controlled intervention studies

The available intervention studies examine the impact of a variety of milk products on circulating cholesterol levels. No evidence exists to suggest that the SFA in milk is deleterious with respect to blood cholesterol. In contrast available data suggest that an as yet unidentified component may exist in milk which may actually confer cardio protection by reducing blood cholesterol levels. In a multi-centred, randomised, controlled intervention trial Barr, McCarron, Heaney, Dawson-Hughes, Berga, Stern and Oparil (2000) examined the impact of 3 glasses (3x 230ml) of either skimmed or semi-skimmed milk per day for 12 weeks adults. No significant effects of milk supplementation on total cholesterol or LDL-cholesterol, either between the control and the milk-supplemented group or in the milk group over time (pre versus post-milk) was evident. In a study published in 1992 (Buonopane, Kilara, Smith and McCarthy,

1992), a significant decrease in total cholesterol levels were evident in individuals with a baseline cholesterol >4.9mmol/l following the consumption of one quart of skimmed milk per day for 8 weeks. This finding would mean that this potentially favourable effect of milk would be available to nearly all but a few milk drinkers, since up to 60% of adults in the UK will have cholesterol above this level. In addition a reduction in blood pressure was evident in the group as a whole.

In conclusion the studies to date conclude that milk, whether whole or skimmed may bring about a modest reduction in total- and LDL-cholesterol. There have been a number of different mediators suggested including magnesium, orotic acid, IgG, riboflavin and an indirect effect via alteration in the gut microflora. However the beneficial component remains largely elusive.

Fermented milk products and cholesterol

The benefits of fermented milk products with respect to cholesterol concentrations was first identified in the Maasai people in Africa, who despite the atherogenic diet have a low incidence of CHD and circulating cholesterol. The cardioprotection has been attributed to a large consumption of fermented milk. A number of recent studies have also suggested that fermented milk products may confer additional benefits when compared to the native milk. In a study where the effect of a yoghurt fermented with either *E. faecium* and 2 strains of *S. thermophilus* was studied to determine the possible hypercholesterolaemic properties a significant reduction in total- and LDL-cholesterol was evident in the test group relative to placebo product which had been acidified using an organic acid (Agerbaeck, Gerdes and Richelsen, 1995). These findings have been confirmed in other studies (St-Onge, Farnworth and Jones, 2000). The proposed mechanism is that the consumption of the probiotic product results in a beneficial effect on the gut bacterial content. This is thought to reduce cholesterol levels either by an alteration in the short chain fatty acid (acetate, propionate and butyrate) production by the gut microflora or by a decongugation of bile salts resulting in increased cholesterol excretion thereby lowering body cholesterol reserves. Short chain fatty acids synthesised in the gut are rapidly absorbed from the large gut and are metabolised by the liver, where they influence cholesterol synthesis and metabolism.

Immunized milk and cholesterol

A limited number of studies have demonstrated the hypocholesterolaemic benefits of milk from immunized cows. The impact of the consumption of 0.3-0.5L/day of skimmed milk from immunized cows versus standard skimmed milk for 8 weeks on blood cholesterol was determined in mildly hypercholesterolaemic adults (Golay, Ferrara, Felber and Schneider, 1990). Significant reduction in total and LDL cholesterol were evident in the immunized milk relative to the control. The proposed mechanism of action is similar to that of fermented milk in that immunized milk may have a beneficial effect on the gastrointestinal flora which may result in additional cholesterol excretion in the faeces (St-Onge, Farnworth and Jones, 2000).

Manipulation of the fatty acid profile of milk

Against a background of general lack of acceptability of a reduced fat diet in the UK and many other countries, and with a much expanded knowledge of the impact of individual fatty acids on blood lipids levels, the focus of dietary guidelines has shifted from recommendations of total fat intake to a greater emphasis on the fatty acid profile of the diet as a means of reducing CHD risk (COMA, 1994). Although milk makes a relatively small contribution to saturated fat intake in the UK, dairy products as a whole currently contribute up to 40%. In view of this focus on the fat composition, much recent research has focussed on improving the fatty acid profile of milk either by manipulation of the diet of the animal or post production alterations in fat content.

Although altering the dietary fatty acid composition of the diet of the animal offers great potential for altering fatty acid intake at a population level, a consensus of the impact of such modification on the welfare of the animal, milk yield and milk fat content, the organoleptic quality and stability of the milk, and on the *trans* fatty acid profile of the milk is currently lacking (see chapter 5). In addition the cost-benefit of such often-expensive dietary manipulation need to be considered. However some successful modifications have been achieved.

Decreasing saturated fatty acids

Long chain fatty acids are potent inhibitors of mammary fatty acid synthesis through a direct inhibitory effect of *de novo* synthesis, resulting in a lower C4:0-C16:0 synthesis, and due to a greater supply of unsaturated fatty acids to the mammary tissue. For example, Mattos and Palmquist (1974) achieved a 40% decrease in C4:0-C16:0 fatty acid on supplementing the cows diet with encapsulated soya oil. Much more modest reductions are observed when the unsaturated oils are fed in the unprotected form.

Increasing polyunsatured fatty acids

PUFA are not synthesised by ruminant tissues. Therefore, the PUFA concentration in milk is dependent on the dietary amount, which flows through the rumen. Feeding encapsulated rapeseed, sunflower, soyabean or cotton seed oil results in an increase in linoleic acid content of milk fat from about 2% to 15-20% (Chilliard, Ferlay, Mansbridge and Doreau, 2000). With diets enriched with unprotected oils or seeds from soyabean or sunflower, the percentage of linoleic acid in milk fat does not increase above 4%. As described for linoleic acid, a significant increase in the linolenic acid content of milk is possible using efficiently protected linseed oil.

Increasing EPA and DHA

An increase in EPA and DHA of up to 2% of total fatty acids can be achieved following protected fish oil feeding, with a increase up to about 1% of total fatty acids following unprotected fish oil feeding (Demeyer and Doreau, 1999; Chilliard *et al*, 2000).

The potential public health benefits of such fatty acid manipulations were demonstrated in a recent study where the SFA:MUFA ratio of milk and meat products was reduced by altering the fatty acid composition of the animal's diet. Dairy products produced using this approach have been shown resulted in a significant reduction in cholesterol levels when fed to human volunteers (Noakes, Nestel and Clifton, 1996), thus highlighting the potential that newly developing animal feeding knowledge and technology could have on reducing population cholesterol levels.

Conclusion

At a population level modest consumption of milk should be encouraged unless a particular allergy to milk components exists. Milk and dairy products represent the main dietary source of calcium. Calcium intake during the first 3 decades of life is one of the most important factors which determines risk of developing osteoporosis later in life. Also a consistent body of animal and cell culture studies suggest that milk products contain an array of anti-carcinogenic components. However efficacy in humans remains to be established.

The view that milk and dairy products have a negative impact on heart disease hinges historically on the inter-relationships between serum cholesterol saturated fat and CHD. This view is not supported by the existing evidence, either from epidemiological data or intervention trials.

In fact milk, and in particular fermented milk products have been shown to result in modest benefits in the blood lipid profile. It must be concluded that a change in the pattern of consumption of milk and dairy products is unlikely to confer significantly negative effects on CHD.

References

Agerbaeck, M., Gerdes, L.U. and Richelsen, B. (1995) Hypocholesterolaemic effect of a new feremnted milk product in middle-aged men. *European Journal of Clinical Nutrition*, **49**, 346-352.

Anitshkow, N. (1913) Changes in the rabbit aorta due to experimentally induced cholesterolsteatosis. Beitrage zur pathologishen Anatomieund zur allgemeinen *Pathologie*, **56**, 379-404.

Barr, S.I., McCarron, D.A., Heaney, R.P., Dawson-Hughes, B., Berga, S.L., Stern, J.S. and Oparil, S. (2000) Effects of increased consumption of fluid milk on energy and nutrient intake, body weight, and cardiovascular risk factors in healthy older adults. *Journal of American Dietetic Association*, **100**, 810-817.

Buonopane, G.J., Kilara, A., Smith, J.S. and McCarthy, R.D. (1992) Effect of skim milk supplementation on blood cholesterol concentration, blood pressure, and triglycerides in a free-living human population. *Journal of the American College of Nutrition*, **11**, 56-67.

Chilliard, Y., Ferlay, A., Mansbridge, R.M. and Doreau, M. (2000) Ruminant milk fat plasticity: nutritional control of saturated, polyunsaturated, *trans* and conjugated fatty acids. *Annals of Zootechnology*, **49**,181-205.

Committee on Medical Aspects of Food Policy (COMA) (1994) Nutritional Aspects of Cardiovascular Disease. Report on Health and Social Subjects No 46. London: HMSO.

Demeyer, D. and Doreau, M. (1999) Targets and procedures for altering ruminant meat and milk. *Proceedings of the Nutrition Society*, **58**, 593-607.

Golay, A., Ferrara, J.M., Felber, J.P. and Schneider, H.(1990) Cholesterol-lowering effect of skim milk from immunized cows in hypercholesterolaemic patients. *American Journal of Clinical Nutrition*, **52**, 1014-1019.

Ha, Y.L., Storkson, J. and Pariza, M.W. (1990) Inhibition of benzo(a)pyrene-induced mouse forestomach neoplasia by conjugated dienoic derivatives of linoleic acid. *Cancer Research*, **50**, 1097-1101.

Hegsted, D.M., Ausman, L.M., Johnson, J.A. and Dallal, G.E. (1993) Dietary fat and serum lipids an evaluation of the experimental data. *American Journal of Clinical Nutrition*, **57**, 875-883.

Hokanson, J. and Austin, M.A. (1996) Plasma triglyceride level is a risk factor for cardiovascular disease independent of high-density lipoprotein cholesterol. *Journal of Cardiovascular Risk*, 3, 213-219.

Hu, F.B., Rimm, E.B., Stampfer, M.J., Ascherio, A., Spiegelman, D. and Willett, W.C. (2000) Prospective study of major dietary patterns and risk of coronary heart disease in men. *American Journal of Clinical Nutrition*, 72, 912-921.

Keys, A., Anderson, J.T. and Grande, F. (1965) Serum cholesterol responses to changes in diet: Particular saturated fatty acids in the diet. *Metabolism*, 14, 776-787.

Knekt, P., Jarvinen, R., Seppanen, R., Pukkala, E. and Aromaa, A.(1996) Intake of dairy products and the risk of breast cancer. *British Journal of Cancer*, 73, 687-691.

Kritchevsky, D., Tepper, S.A., Wright, S., Tso, P. and Czarnecki, S.K. (2000) Influence of conjugated linoleic acid (CLA) on establishment and progression of atherosclerosis in rabbits. *Journal of American Colleges of Nutrition*, 19, 472S-477S

Mattos, W. and Palmquist, D.L. (1974) Increasing polyunsaturated fatty acid yields in milk of cows fed protected fat. *Journal of Dairy Science*, 57, 1050-1054.

McCance and Widdowson (1998) The Composition of Foods: Fatty Acid supplement. London: HMSO.

Menotti, A., Kromhout, D., Blackburn, H., Fidanza, F, Buzina, R., Nissinen, A (1999) Food intake patterns and 25-year mortality from coronary heart disease:cross cultural correlations in the Seven Countries Study. The Seven Countries Study Research Group. *European Journal of Epidemiology*, 15, 507-515

Mensink, R.P. and Katan, M.B. (1992) Effect of dietary fatty acids on serum lipids and lipoproteins. A meta-analysis of 27 trials. *Arteriosclerosis and Thrombosis*, 12, 911-919.

Mensink, R.P. and Zock, P.L. (1998) Lipoprotein metabolism and trans fatty acids. *In*: Sebedio, J.L. and Christie, W.W. (eds.). Dundee, The Oily Press.

Minihane, A.M., Khan, S., Leigh-Firbank, E.C., Talmud, P., Wright, J.W., Murphy, M.C., Griffin, B.A. and Williams, C.M. (2000) ApoE polymorphism and fish oil supplementation in subjects with an atherogenic lipoprotein phenotype (ALP). *Arteriosclerosis, Thrombosis and Vascular Biology*, 20, 1990-1997.

Ness, A.R., Smith, G.D. and Hart, C. (2001) Milk coronary heart disease and mortality. *Journal of Epidemiology and Community Health*, 55, 379-382.

Noakes, M., Nestel, P.J. and Clifton, P.M. (1996) Modifying the fatty acid profile of dairy products through feedlot technology lowers plasma cholesterol of human consuming the products. *American Journal of Clinical Nutrition*, 63, 42-46.

Office for National Statistics. 2001. Available from www.statistics.gov.uk.

Scandinavian Simvastatin Survival Study Group (1994) Randomised trial of cholesterol lowering in 4444 patients with coronary heart disease: the Scandinavian Simvastatin Survival Study (4S). *Lancet*, 344, 1383-1389.

Shepherd, J., Cobbe, S.M., Ford, I., Isles, C.G., Lorimer, A.R., MacFarlane, P.W. and Packard, C.J. (1995) Prevention of coronary heart disease with pravastatin in men with hypercholesterolaemia. *New England Journal of Medicine*, 333, 1301-1307.

St-Onge, M.P., Farnworth, E.R. and Jones, P.J.H (2000) Consumption of fermented and non-fermented dairy products: effects on cholesterol concentrations and metabolism. *American Journal of Clinical Nutrition*, 71, 674-681.

Willett, W.C., Stampfer, M.J., Manson, J.E., Colditz, G.A., Speizer, F.E., Rosner, B.A., Sampson, L.A. and Hennekens, C.H. (1993) Intake of trans fatty acids and risk of coronary heart disease among women. *The Lancet*, 341, 581-585.

Williams, C.M. (2000). Dietary fatty acids and human health. *Annals of Zootechnology*, 49, 165-180.

Index